Developing Online Learning Environments in Nursing Education

Third Edition

Carol A. O'Neil, PhD, RN, CNE, is an Associate Professor at the University of Maryland School of Nursing. She is Co-director of the Institute for Educators in Nursing and Health Professions and teaches in its online teaching certificate program. Dr. O'Neil is a Web Initiative in Teaching (WIT) Fellow, an initiative supported by the University System of Maryland. In addition to two previous editions of this book, she has a journal article, book chapter, and many national and international presentations related to teaching in online environments.

Cheryl A. Fisher, EdD, RN-BC, is currently the Senior Nurse Consultant for Extramural Collaborations at the National Institutes of Health in Bethesda, Maryland, serving as a resource to the extramural sites outside of the Clinical Center conducting clinical research. Formerly she was the Program Director for Professional Development with a staff of eight nursing education specialists. She has also been an adjunct faculty with the University of Maryland, teaching online graduate and undergraduate courses in nursing informatics for the past 10 years and holds a doctorate in Instructional Technology from Towson University.

Matthew J. Rietschel, MS, is the Director of Educational Strategies in the Office of Learning Technologies at the University of Maryland School of Nursing. Mr. Rietschel is the Director of Learning Technologies and a clinical instructor at the University of Maryland School of Nursing. He received his bachelor's in education from Salisbury University and his master's in instructional technology from Towson University where he is currently working on his doctorate in instructional technology. He currently supervises the development and deployment of all web-based and blended courses, supports a multitude of grant projects involving technology, and teaches in the Teaching in Nursing and Health Professions Certificate program.

Developing Online Learning Environments in Nursing Education

Third Edition

Carol A. O'Neil, PhD, RN, CNE

Cheryl A. Fisher, EdD, RN-BC

Matthew J. Rietschel, MS

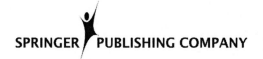

SPRINGER PUBLISHING COMPANY

Springer Publishing Company, LLC
11 West 42nd Street
New York, NY 10036
www.springerpub.com

Acquisitions Editor: Joe Morita
Composition: Amnet

ISBN: 978-0-8261-9913-3
e-book ISBN: 978-0-8261-9914-0

13 14 15 16/5 4 3 2 1

The author and the publisher of this Work have made every effort to use sources believed to be reliable to provide information that is accurate and compatible with the standards generally accepted at the time of publication. The author and publisher shall not be liable for any special, consequential, or exemplary damages resulting, in whole or in part, from the readers' use of, or reliance on, the information contained in this book. The publisher has no responsibility for the persistence or accuracy of URLs for external or third-party Internet websites referred to in this publication and does not guarantee that any content on such websites is, or will remain, accurate or appropriate.

Library of Congress Cataloging-in-Publication Data

O'Neil, Carol A.
    Developing online learning environments in nursing education / Carol A. O'Neil, Cheryl A. Fisher, Matthew J. Rietschel. – 3rd ed.
      p. ; cm.
    Includes bibliographical references and index.
    ISBN 978-0-8261-9913-3 (alk. paper) – ISBN 978-0-8261-9914-0 (e-book)
    I. Fisher, Cheryl A. II. Rietschel, Matthew J. III. Title.
    [DNLM: 1. Education, Nursing–methods. 2. Curriculum. 3. Education, Distance. 4. Internet. WY 18]
    RT73
    610.73071'1–dc23
                                                                    2013009312

Printed in the United States of America by Gasch Printing.

We dedicate this book to our spouses, children, and grandchildren, who have supported us to persevere with our commitment to online education.

Contents

Contributors

Susan Bindon, DNP, RN-BC, is an Assistant Professor at the University of Maryland School of Nursing, teaching online graduate courses in nursing education. She has 20 years of nursing education experience in academic and staff development settings, and in classroom, clinical, and online learning environments. She was Director of Education at a Baltimore-area health system where she was responsible for the competency and continuing education of clinical staff and had oversight for the organization's learning management system. Dr. Bindon is active in the Association for Nursing Professional Development and is currently serving a 2-year term on the Board of Directors. She has served 5 years on the Editorial Board for the *Journal for Nurses in Staff Development (JNSD)* and acted as *JNSD*'s Website Editor as well. Dr. Bindon is ANCC certified in Nursing Professional Development, and is a review course instructor for ANCC's Nursing Professional Development certification exam.

Kathleen M. Buckley, PhD, RN, IBCLC, is an Associate Professor in the School of Nursing at the University of Maryland, where she has been a key player in transitioning the Doctor of Nursing Practice program from a traditional face-to-face format to a blended hybrid learning format. She has expertise in the use of web conferencing for instructional purposes and plays a major role in training the school's faculty and students in the use of these technologies. Dr. Buckley is also certified as a Master Reviewer for *Quality Matters*, a leader in quality assurance for online education, and has participated as an external reviewer for a number of online and blended nursing courses throughout the United States.

Kathleen A. Gould, RD, MA, LDN, is a Clinical Assistant Professor in the Department of Health Science at Towson University. She is pursuing her doctorate in instructional technology at Towson University with a concentration in online learning. Ms. Gould has experience teaching online and implementing problem-based learning in this environment. Her doctoral research is focused on student self-directed learning readiness and success in online problem-based learning.

William A. Sadera, PhD, is Professor of Instructional Technology at Towson University. Dr. Sadera currently serves as the Director of the Doctoral Program in Instructional Technology in Towson University's College of Education. He has been active in the field of Instructional Technology and Online Learning, having taught courses, conducted research projects, and published on these topics for over 15 years; his current research focuses on online professional development, pedagogy, and effective design of online instruction.

Special thanks to **Sheila Prados** for her research and resource gathering that supports best practices throughout this book.

Preface

Four years have passed since the last edition of our book, and the current status report is: Some things are the same and some things are different!

The things that are the same are areas of reconceptualization, design, infrastructure, interaction, and managing and evaluating courses. There are more articles available in the literature that provide evidence for best practices in teaching and learning online. These best practices have been included in this current edition.

The things that are different include the technology and the increased specialization among nursing educators. Technology is being used by nursing educators to guide students in making smarter choices for best practices and better outcomes. These choices are now available via portable and smaller devices as well as mobile apps and tablets.

Nursing students are tech savvy and come to nursing school with the expectation of using technology. Students take courses online and in blended learning environments. Most courses are now blended to some degree, even if only the syllabus and resources are online. Students are learning from mobile apps, Web 2.0 tools, and streaming videos in the skills laboratory and in simulation labs with high fidelity equipment.

Students graduate and begin lifelong learning. Orientation to their first nursing job will include mobile apps and simulations and using the technology that was introduced in school. The focus is different in that what they learn in orientation now impacts how they will care for patients.

Learning has become more specialized, especially in teaching patients. There are diabetic educators, wound care educators, and others, and the field of patient education has now moved beyond a chapter in a book such as that included in the last edition and has now become a book unto itself.

More literature is coming from nursing professional development educators, and this area of education is beginning to grow. Teaching students is still the goal of nursing education, but the focus is changing to transitional programs in schools of nursing to patient care environments. Hospital educators and nursing educators are talking and sharing ideas of how to prepare nurses to leave school and enter the work force. Education is seen as lifelong learning and thus the focus of this book is on teaching students and professional development.

What is on the horizon?

We would be remiss in not mentioning the current trend of the Massive Online Open Course (MOOC). Started about 4 years ago with a course that was free, the MOOC consists of courses open to registrants beyond their school. The professors are well known for the universities at which they teach and for their fields of expertise. The students enroll because they have an interest in learning from the experts.

Two major technology and education reports in January, 2013, describe the MOOC as an emerging concept that has the potential for changing the current landscape of both traditional and online education as we know it today. Students go to the website and enroll in courses with large numbers of fellow students (in the thousands). They use current technology to meet the course objectives, are evaluated, receive grades, and are issued a certificate. The method is there but how it will impact the educational system in the future is yet to be determined. Stay tuned for more developments in this widely popular movement.

This book is still about using the web and all its richness to teach students and professional nurses how to use technology and to maintain competency and embrace lifelong learning as a nursing professional. The nurses performing these activities need knowledge and skills such as pedagogy and the study of learning, specifically learning through a guided constructivist model (Chapter 2); the infrastructure needed to facilitate online strategies (Chapter 3); the technology courseware and software necessary to teach in online environments (Chapter 4); reconceptualizing course content from face-to-face to an online environment (Chapter 5); designing online learning environments (Chapter 6); creating blended-learning environments (Chapter 7);

communicating and interacting online (Chapter 8); managing online learning (Chapter 9); assessing and evaluating learning in online environments (Chapter 10); the theory of continuing medical education (Chapter 11); and preparing for professional staff development (Chapter 12).

We hope you enjoy the practicality of this book and have fun in the process!

Carol A. O'Neil
Cheryl A. Fisher
Matthew J. Rietschel

ONE

Introduction to Teaching and Learning in Online Environments

CAROL A. O'NEIL

The purpose of this chapter is to present the history and to introduce the basic concepts of learning in online environments. When the learner and the teacher are separated by geography and time, the learning is called "distance learning" (Williams, Paprock, & Covington, 1999). The Sloan Consortium (Allen & Seaman, 2013) defines online learning in terms of the proportion of content that is delivered online: When 80% or more of the content is delivered online, the course is called an online course. When 30% to 79% is online, the course is called hybrid or blended. When only 1% to 29% of the content is online, the course is described as web facilitated, and when no part of the course is online, it is called a traditional class.

Online learning is instructor moderated, instructor taught, and instructor mentored, yet student self-directed. An online learning environment can comprise large discussion groups, small group discussions, individual activities, group activities, and various levels of interaction between and among students, faculty, and the content. Content can be presented in a variety of ways, including video casting, audio taping, films, and links to the web, charts, graphs, statistical data, formulas, and case studies. Interaction can be synchronous (real time) or asynchronous (delayed). Synchronous interaction means having a live discussion online where the faculty can be seen and students and faculty can hear and/or see each other. Asynchronous communication entails leaving messages at specific posting sites that others in the learning environment can read at their convenience, such as discussion boards, blogs, and wikis.

Individual courses, groups of courses, and entire programs can be offered online. The degree of Internet use in a course ranges from supplementing classroom learning to courses and programs that are offered completely online. Online learners can attend traditional universities, such as Pennsylvania State University (www.worldcampus.psu.edu), or virtual universities, such as California Virtual University (www.cvc.edu). In addition to online courses and programs, online journals are available that focus on teaching and learning online, such as the *Journal of Asynchronous Learning Networks*. There are professional organizations that provide resources for online teaching and learning such as EDUCAUSE (www.educause.edu) and the Sloan Consortium (http://sloanconsortium.org/). Some courses can be taken online free of charge at web sites such as Coursera (https://www.coursera.org).

HISTORICAL PERSPECTIVE OF TEACHING WITH TECHNOLOGY

Teaching and learning at a distance in not new to education. Paper-based distance curricula in which learners enrolled in universities and received their learning packages in the mail have been available for some time. Early correspondence courses enabled learners and instructors to interact, although with a significant time lag between message production and reception (Woods & Baker, 2004). Television has also provided a medium for teaching and learning at a distance. Students in remote areas could use the television to obtain learning content. In the late 1960s, Schramm (1962) conducted studies that compared instructional television (ITV) with classroom instruction and summarized the results of more than 400 empirical studies. The findings of his research were that there is no significant difference between learning from a television or from a classroom.

As distance education progressed from correspondence courses to online learning, opportunities for interpersonal interaction also increased. Videoconferencing made it possible for learners and faculty to interact in real time. With the emergence of the Internet, particularly email and the World Wide Web, it became possible to promote high degrees of interaction utilizing mainstream technology and cost-effective learning environments.

Following Schramm's (1962) conclusions that there was no significant difference in learning between the traditional classroom and televised learning, researchers compared classroom instruction to other methods of distance education. Numerous studies comparing traditional classroom–based instruction with technology-supported instruction have found no significant difference in critical educational variables, such as learning outcomes. Wetzel, Radtke, and Stern (1994) summarized the results of comparative studies conducted through the mid-1990s and also found no significant differences in learning outcomes between the two learning environments. Thomas Russell (1999) at North Carolina State University studied hundreds of sources of written material about distance education and concluded that the learning outcomes of students in the traditional classroom are similar to those of students in distance technology classes. This was termed the *no significant differences phenomenon.*

The American Federation of Teachers and the National Education Association commissioned The Institute of Higher Education Policy to conduct a review of the current research on the effectiveness of distance education (Merisotis & Phipps, 1999). Merisotis and Phipps (1999) reviewed studies published in the 1990s and published "What's the Difference: A Review of Contemporary Research on the Effectiveness of Distance Learning in Education." The findings were that students online tend to perform as effectively as traditional students. Online students had similar learning experiences and were as satisfied with their learning experiences as traditional students. But the authors noted several shortcomings in the original research: lack of control for extraneous variables, lack of randomization of subjects, questionable validity and reliability of instruments used to measure student outcome and attitude, and no control for reactive effects such as the impact of motivation and interest because taking a course online is a novelty. The authors suggest that because of these shortcomings, the study was inconclusive. The question—what is the best way to teach students—prevailed (Merisotis & Phipps, 1999).

Other variables were then studied, including overall course satisfaction, course organization, and meeting class objectives. Leasure, Davis, and Thievon (2000) looked at these variables in traditional lecture and distance-based instruction and reported no significant differences. Course satisfaction was evaluated by Allen, Bourhis, and Mabry (2002). These authors conducted a meta-analysis and found no differences in satisfaction levels but found a slight preference for traditional face-to-face courses over distance-based education courses. Researchers began to move beyond comparative studies and into other methods, such as discourse analysis and in-depth interviews. These methods have provided theoretical frameworks on which to base various studies and have revealed further complexities involved in distance education, such as social, economic, and global issues affecting the field (Saba, 2000).

Chickering and Ehrman (1966) used the American Association for Higher Education (AAHE) Principles for Good Practice to develop best practices to teach students in online environments and developed a paper called "Implementing the Seven Principles: Technology as Lever." The following points are the best practices and examples.

1. *Good practice encourages contact between students and faculty.*
   Students and faculty exchange thoughts and ideas more effectively and safely in online environments than in the traditional classroom. Communication becomes more intimate, protected, and connected in online rather than in face-to-face interaction.
2. *Good practice develops reciprocity and cooperation among students.*
   Technology provides opportunities for interaction in online learning environments. Students can share their knowledge and experiences in small groups, in study groups, during group problem-solving exercises, and in activities related to learning content. For example, the learning content may be epidemiology and the epidemiologic triangle: the agent, the host, and the environment. Online students can be assigned to small learning groups and given the assignment to explain how West Nile virus occurs and suggest strategies to prevent it from occurring.
3. *Good practice uses active learning techniques.*
   The technology included in online learning systems provides opportunity for active learning. For example, students in an online

community health nursing course are given an exercise to assess a community. Students are directed to obtain census and vital statistics data. Students then view a windshield survey (made by the faculty). The exercise is to use both of these sources of information to write a composite picture of the community to share with their learning group. The group consensus summary is posted in a public discussion forum for all groups to read.

4. *Good practice gives prompt feedback.*
   Technology provides many opportunities for feedback, both synchronous (real time), asynchronous (time delayed), and via email. What is to be considered "prompt" should be defined in the course directions or in the syllabus. For example, the instructor might post the following message: "I will read all postings on the discussion board and post a comment to the group at the end of the week." Or the faculty might post "I will answer all emails within 3 working days."

5. *Good practice emphasizes time on task.*
   Time is critical and using time wisely is important. Online courses save the students commuting time and parking costs. Students can learn anywhere—at home, at work, or virtually anywhere there is an Internet connection. A rule of thumb to determine the number of hours a week that students will spend on an online course is to double or triple the number of course credits. For example, a student enrolled in a 3-credit course can expect to spend 6 to 9 hours each week working on the course.

6. *Good practice communicates high expectations.*
   Some students register for online courses because they think they will be easier than traditional courses. They soon find out that this is a fallacy. Expectations should be clearly communicated to students. If students are not performing at the expected level, the faculty should email the student and describe observed behavior and delineate expected behavior. For example, if the faculty sees that a student is posting such comments as "I agree" or "Great idea" the faculty should send a feedback email to this student saying, "I have read your postings and can see that in some you clearly express your ideas and use the literature to support your ideas, but in other postings your comments are less substantiated. I can see that you have excellent ideas and would like to see you share these more with your peers."

7. *Good practice respects diverse talents and ways of learning.* The advantage of online courses is the many resources available to accommodate a variety of learning styles. For example, for the visual learners, use PowerPoint and charts and graphs. For audio learners, use podcasts. For readers, add notes. Slide presentations can be easily constructed for disseminating content online. Links to YouTube videos and a plethora of websites can be added to the slides.

Billings and Connors (n.d.) applied these best practices to nursing. They suggest a model that focuses on the best practices for technology, faculty, students, and outcomes. They developed a set of examples for each of the areas of focus in the model. For example, a best practice for technology is infrastructure, and the evidence includes access to the internet, course management software, user support, and appropriate hardware and software.

While the guiding principles of quality practice were being developed, universities were struggling with what Noble (1998) calls automation. According to Noble, automation, "the distribution of digitized course material online, without the participation of professors who develop such material—is often justified as an inevitable part of the new knowledge based society" (Noble, 1998, p. 1). University of California at Los Angeles (UCLA) instituted the "Instructional Enhancement Initiative," which mandated that all Arts and Sciences courses have a web-based delivery component. The university partnered with private corporations and formed its own for-profit company (Noble, 1998). Noble says "it is by no accident that the high tech transformation of higher education is being initiated and implemented from the top down, either without any student and faculty involvement in the decision making or despite it" (Noble, 1998, p. 2). Although faculty and students were opposed to the initiative, UCLA administrators continued with their plans (Noble, 1998). Further, Noble cites a reason for the decision to continue—the fear of being left behind in an academic trend. He calls this "the commercialism of higher education" (Noble, 1998). The function of the university is to teach and universities are developing their courseware into marketable, sellable products in hopes of getting "a piece of the commercial action for their institutions or themselves, as vendors in their own right of software and content" (Noble, 1998, p. 5). The concern of faculty is the quality of education. Faculty view web-based instruction as commoditizing education and the fear is that the quality of instruction will be compromised by automation.

Online courses and programs grew from 1999 to 2001 through grants awarded by the Department of Education called "Learning Anytime Anywhere Partnerships" (LAAP) for innovative distance learning projects that included partnerships. With funding from President Bill Clinton's Fund for the Improvement of Postsecondary Education, LAAP received $10 million in 1999, $23.3 million in 2000, and $30 million in 2001. The project was phased out but the emphasis on partnerships in projects continued to grow (Carnevale, 2001).

CURRENT STATE OF ONLINE LEARNING

The U.S. Census Bureau (2010) has included questions about computer use in their census surveys since 1984 and Internet use since 1997. They report that 81.4% of U.S. households had computers and 75.9% of the population lived in a household with Internet access in 2010. What are people doing online? Approximately 11% are taking courses online; 35% are searching about health care; 33% are searching government services; and 35% are searching for employment.

How are computers being used in teaching and learning? Campus Computing is the largest continuing study of the role of computing and information technology in American higher education. Their 2012 survey provided data from 2,800 public and private colleges and universities throughout the United States (Allen & Seaman, 2013). The focus of online learning in their 2013 report is on Massive Open Online Courses (MOOCs). A consortium of colleges and universities come together and offer their courses online for no fee. An example is Coursera (https://www.coursera.org). What is under discussion is how MOOCs will impact education. Allen and Seaman (2013) reported on the status of online education in 2012. They report that 77% of chief academic officers in the colleges and universities they surveyed think that online learning is superior to or better than classroom learning. They report that 6.7 million students were enrolled in at least one online course and 32% of students now take at least one course online. Faculty are not as positive about online courses and this has been a steady trend over the past several years.

The Horizon Report (EDUCAUSE, 2012) is an annual report that describes emerging technologies that will most likely impact education online. They suggest technologies to watch in the next 12 months, 2 to 3 years, and 4 to 5 years. The 2012 technologies that have emerged are mobile apps and tablet computing. In the next 2 to 3 years, the report suggests the focus will change to game-based learning and learning analytics. Technologies to watch over the next 4 to 5 years are gesture-based computing and the Internet of things. Things are smart objects; one example is a micro camera that is ingested and is used for diagnostic testing. The short list of findings of the 2013 Horizon Report were released (EDUCAUSE, 2013). Technology to be watched in the next year are flipped classrooms (blended courses in which content is online and active learning takes place in the classroom), MOOCs, mobile apps, and tablet computing. The 2 to 3 year time to adoption technologies are the same as those for 2012 with the addition of augmented reality (called blended reality). The 4 to 5 year time to adoption includes 3D printing, flexible displays, next-generation batteries and wearable technology (EDUCAUSE, 2013).

More web 2.0 tools such as blogs and wikis will be used and learning will be a collective experience of ideas and knowledge. Boundaries will be more fluid and technology will be smaller and more powerful. It is estimated that about 70% of academic learners believe that student demand for online learning is still growing and about 83% of institutions who currently offer courses online think that their enrollments in online courses will increase (Allen & Seaman, 2007).

ONLINE AND TRADITIONAL LEARNING ENVIRONMENTS

What are the differences between online and traditional or face-to-face learning environments? The online learning environment is accessible anytime and anywhere, which makes it convenient for the learner. Online learning is dependent only on technology: If the technology is available, so is the education. Traditional learning is scheduled, and classes are offered at set times in specific places. The course a learner needs may only be offered 50 miles away at 8 a.m. The student must be available when and where the course is offered. Traditional learning tends to be a one-size-fits-all approach, with lecture as the major teaching modality.

In an online learning environment, students can log on and review their course material whenever they want and wherever a computer with Internet access is available. Online students are spared driving to class during the winter months in snowy locations. They are also spared the inconvenience of traffic, the scarcity and cost of parking, and the worry of compromised safety, especially when taking night classes in cities.

Because learning online is technology dependent, the GIGO rule applies: Garbage-In, Garbage-Out. Online learning is not merely "slapping classroom content online." Rather, the positive resources of technology are used to bring content and experiences to learners. In other words, the resource is used to enrich the content. Learning online can be seen as a lonely and isolated experience and that is because online learners cannot see each other, and their teacher cannot see the students. "If you can't see them, you can't teach them," seems to be a traditionalist mantra. Getting back to GIGO, online education that excludes interaction denies the learner a quality learning experience. Online learners should be actively interacting with each other (student to student), with the teacher (student to teacher), and with the content (student to content).

The American Academy (2007–2012) offers 10 advantages of taking online courses. The first is that online learning is flexible and will fit the student's schedule and pace of learning and students can work on the course anywhere (with a computer and Internet connection). Online courses save time and money in driving and parking costs, may be more budget friendly and eliminate the need for a dress code. Content can be reviewed over and over. There is more time for other pursuits or responsibilities; it develops self-control and commitment and allows the student to plan ahead. The only caveat is that the student will need self-discipline and a sense of responsibility.

CHARACTERISTICS OF AN ONLINE COURSE

An online course consists of an audience, a purpose, learning objectives, content, design, interaction, and assessment and evaluation activities. In an online learning module, there are objectives that tell learners what they will accomplish in the course. In addition, orientation and support services are provided for teachers and learners. A learning module should be about 60% self-study and 40% interaction. The format for the learner is to read the material, do the activities and assignments, discuss the content, and report on assignments.

Characteristics of an effective online course or program include an effective course structure and design, engaging learning activities, interaction, and effective assessment strategies (Education.com, 2006–2013). A successful course is planned and well thought out. It includes active learning strategies that require participation and use of the literature to support ideas. Interaction should move to creating a learning community in which students and faculty feel connected with one other and with their learning. Assessment strategies should consider alternative and traditional testing.

SUCCESSFUL ONLINE STUDENTS

The Illinois Online Network (2010) suggests that students who most benefit from online learning live long distances from the campus and have busy lives with families, a profession, and other responsibilities. The successful student is mature, open-minded, self-motivated, accepting of critical thinking, and willing to work collaboratively, with good written communication skills and a minimum level of technology experience. Successful online students (Pedagogy and Learning, 2010) should have these qualities:

- Be open minded about sharing knowledge and experience
- Be able to communicate effectively in writing
- Be self-motivated and self-disciplined
- Have access to a computer
- Be able to think before responding
- Value the quality of learning online

CHARACTERISTICS OF SUCCESSFUL FACULTY

The Illinois Online Network (Pedagogy and Learning, 2012) describes basic criteria for an online facilitator. The facilitator should have a broad base of life experiences including how to translate learning to the real world. The faculty must be sensitive, open, and flexible to facilitate learning in an online environment. Communicating by writing is essential and experience, training, and credentials to teach the content are a must.

Lawrence Ragan (n.d.) suggests 10 principles for faculty. The first is to show up and teach. Faculty facilitate courses and are present to teach and be proactive about and maintain the course management strategies. Faculty create a learning environment that is predictable yet flexible; one that is a quality learning environment with feedback that moves learning in a forward direction. Other characteristics are to provide a safe environment, in which learning is fun and effective.

SUMMARY

Online courses are growing and more courses are offered online and more students are registering for online courses than before. The flexibility of the learning environment is enticing and many learners who would not be able to obtain a degree in traditional educational settings are now able to take courses and earn degrees online. Not all students will be successful online. A successful online student should be comfortable with technology; be self-motivated; and have acceptable writing skills. Not all faculty should teach online. Successful online faculties are flexible facilitators of learning.

REFERENCES

Allen, E., & Seaman, J. (2007). Online nation: Five years of growth in online learning. Babson Survey Research Group and the Sloan Consortium.

Allen, E., & Seaman, J. (2013). Changing course: Ten years of tracking online education in the United States. Retrieved from http://sloanconsortium.org/publications/survey/changing_course_2012

Allen, M., Bourhis, J., Burrell, N., & Mabry, E. (2002). Comparing student satisfaction with distance education to traditional classrooms in higher education: A metaanalysis. *American Journal of Distance Education, 16*(2), 83–97.

American Academy. (2007–2012). Top 10 advantages to taking an online course. Retrieved from http://www.theamericanacademy.com/blog/Taking-Online-Courses-Top-10

Billings, B., & Connors, H. (n.d.). Best practices in online learning. Retrieved from http://www.electronicvision.com/nln/chapter02/

Carnevale, D. (2001, September 28). Education Department cuts new distance education grants. *Chronicle of Higher Education.*

Chickering, A. W., & Ehrmann, S. C. (1966). Implementing the seven principles: Technology as a lever. Retrieved from http://www.tltgroup.org/programs/seven.html

Education.com. (2006–2013). Characteristics of effective distance courses and programs. Retrieved from http://www.education.com/reference/article/effective-distance-courses-program/

EDUCAUSE Learning Initiatives. (2012). 2012 horizon report. Retrieved from http://www.educause.edu/library/resources/2012-horizon-report

EDUCAUSE Learning Initiatives. (2013). NMC horizon project short list 2013 higher education edition. Retrieved from http://www.nmc.org/pdf/2013-horizon-higher-ed-shortlist.pdf

Leasure, A., Davis, L., & Thievon, S. (2000). Comparison of student outcomes and preferences in a traditional vs. World Wide Web–based baccalaureate nursing research course. *Journal of Nursing Education, 39*(4), 149–154.

Merisotis, J. P., & Phipps, R. A. (1999). What's the difference? A review of contemporary research on the effectiveness of distance learning in higher education. Washington, DC: The Institute for Higher Education Policy.

Noble, D. F. (1998). Digital diploma mills: The automation of higher education. Retrieved from http://firstmonday.org/ojs/index.php/fm/article/view/569/490%3E

Pedagogy and Learning. (2010). Illinois online network. Retrieved from http://www.ion.uillinois.edu/resources/tutorials/pedagogy/StudentProfile.asp

Ragan, L. (n.d.). 10 principles of effective online teaching: Best practices in distance education. Retrieved from http://www.eou.edu/~bb/workshops/10%20Principles%20of%20Effective%20Online%20Teaching.pdf

Russell, T. (1999). *No significant difference: A comparative research annotated bibliography on technology for distance education: As reported in 355 research reports, summaries and papers.* Raleigh, NC: North Carolina State University.

Saba, F. (2000). Research in distance education: A status report. *International Review of Research in Open and Distance Learning.* Retrieved April 21, 2008, from http://www.irrodl.org/index.php/irrodl/article/viewArticle/4

Schramm, W. (1962). What we know about learning from instructional television. In *Educational television: The next ten years.* Stanford, CA: The Institute for Commnication Research, Stanford University.

U.S. Census Bureau (2010). Retrieved from www.census.gov

Wetzel, D., Radtke, P., & Stern, H. (1994). *Instructional effectiveness of video media.* Hillsdale, NJ: Lawrence Earlbaum Associates.

Williams, M. L., Paprock, K., & Covington B. (1999). *Distance learning: The essential guide.* London: Sage Publications.

Woods, R., & Baker, J. (2004). Interaction and immediacy in online learning. *International Review of Research in Open and Distance Learning, 5*(2), 1–13.

TWO

Pedagogy Associated With Learning in Online Environments

WILLIAM A. SADERA, CAROL A. O'NEIL,
AND KATHLEEN A. GOULD

Pedagogy is the theory, methods, and activities for maximizing teaching and learning. Bill Pelz (2004) identified the following three principles of effective online pedagogy:

- Principle 1: Let the students do (most of) the work.
- Principle 2: Interactivity is the heart and soul of effective asynchronous learning.
- Principle 3: Strive for presence.

His belief is that the pedagogy of learning online is grounded in student-centered learning and in employing active learning activities. Interactivity is essential for learning online and the presence of both faculty and students is essential for effective online learning. Pedagogy includes the consideration of the influences of developmental level and learning style on learning and the learning theories upon which online learning environments are created.

INFLUENCES ON LEARNING: DEVELOPMENTAL LEVEL

Adult Learning

Online learners are often adults and an effective instructor needs to understand how adults learn. Compared to children and teens, adults have special needs and requirements as learners. Adult learning is not a unique and specific process; rather, it is a set of generalizations about "the adult learner" that imply that students within a certain, yet-to-be-defined age range form a homogeneous group. But differences of culture, cognitive style, life experiences, and gender may be far more important to learning than age (Shannon, 2003).

Malcolm Knowles (1970) pioneered the field of adult learning and identified adult learning characteristics that should be appropriately incorporated into the development of education. Knowles found that adults are autonomous and self-directed. Their teachers must actively involve adult participants in the learning process and serve as facilitators for them. Specifically, instructors must get the participants' perspectives about what topics to cover and let them work on projects that reflect their interests. Instructors should allow the participants to assume responsibility for presentations and group leadership. Instructors have to be sure to act as facilitators, guiding participants to their own knowledge rather than supplying them with facts. Finally, instructors must show participants how the class will help them reach their goals. Adults have accumulated a wealth of life experiences and knowledge that may include work-related activities, family responsibilities, and previous education. Adult learners need to connect learning to this knowledge and experience base. To help them do so, teachers should draw out the participants' experience and knowledge that is relevant to the topic. Educators relate theories and concepts to the participants and recognize the value of experience in learning.

Knowles identified another characteristic of adults: They are goal oriented. Upon enrolling in a course, adult learners usually know what goal they want to attain. Therefore, they appreciate an educational program that is well organized and has clearly defined elements. Instructors must show participants how the class will help them attain these goals and must ensure that the course is relevant and practical. Learning should be applicable to their work or other responsibilities in order for it to be of value to them. In adulthood, learning is best achieved when the subject matter is presented in an authentic learning environment. Instructors must relate the relevance of the lesson to the learner's job or profession. Instructors must show adult learners respect and acknowledge the wealth of experiences these students bring to the classroom. Adult learners should be treated as equals in experience and knowledge and be allowed to voice their opinions freely in class. Because of these characteristics, adult learning programs should capitalize on the experience of the participants, and should adapt to the age range of the participants. Additionally, the course offerings should consider advanced stages of participant development by offering as much choice as possible in the organization of the learning program.

INFLUENCES ON LEARNING: LEARNING STYLE

Learning styles are simply different ways in which we think and learn. Understanding and addressing different learning styles when preparing instructional materials will enhance the entire teaching and learning process. There are many approaches to identifying learning styles. Four methods of assessing learning style are: VARK®, Index of Learning Style, Multiple Intelligences, and the Myers Briggs Type Indicator. The VARK (which standard for visual, aural, read/write, kinesthetic; http://www.varkarn.com/english/index.asp) is a 13-item online questionnaire that provides users with a profile of their visual, auditory, or kinesthetic preferences. "Let me see it!" exemplifies the visual learner; "Just tell me!" exemplifies the auditory learner, and "Let me do it!" is the kinesthetic learner.

The Index of Learning Style (http://www.engr.ncsu.edu/learningstyles/ilsweb.html) is a 44-item online questionnaire that assesses preferences on four dimensions: active/reflective, sensing/intuitive, visual/verbal, and sequential/global. Active learners prefer to apply learning, and reflective learners prefer to think about learning. Sensing learners like to learn facts, while intuitive learners like to learn through discovery. The visual learner learns by seeing, while the verbal learner learns by hearing. Sequential learners are linear and logical and learn in steps, and global learners learn by seeing the big picture first and then seeing the component parts. Howard Gardner, developer of the Multiple Intelligences Theory, describes nine intelligences. Thirteen Online (Educational Broadcasting

Company, 2004) provides an online workshop for "Tapping into Multiple Intelligences" and a comprehensive "Multiple Intelligence Inventory" (with 80 questions). The intelligences and definitions of Gardner's Multiple Intelligences are:

■ Verbal Linguistic Intelligence: well-developed verbal skills and sensitivity to the sounds, meanings, and rhythms of words
■ Mathematical Logical Intelligence: ability to think conceptually and abstractly and capacity to discern logical or numerical patterns
■ Musical Intelligence: ability to produce and appreciate rhythm, pitch, and timber
■ Visual Spatial Intelligence: capacity to think in images and pictures and to visualize accurately and abstractly
■ Bodily Kinesthetic Intelligence: ability to control one's body movements and to handle objects skillfully
■ Interpersonal Intelligence: capacity to detect and respond appropriately to the moods, motivations, and desires of others
■ Intrapersonal Intelligence: capacity to be self-aware and in tune with inner feelings, values, beliefs, and thinking processes
■ Naturalist Intelligence: ability to recognize and categorize plants, animals, and other objects in nature
■ Existential Intelligence: sensitivity and capacity to tackle deep questions about human existence, such as the meaning of life, why do we die, and how did we get here (Educational Broadcasting Company, 2004).

Meacham (2003) suggests characteristics and learning strategies for each of the learning styles, as outlined in Table 2.1. The Myers Briggs Type Indicator (MBTI) is a method of assessing learning style as inferred from a personality inventory. It provides data on four sets of preferences. These preferences result in 16 learning styles, or types. A type is the combination of the four preferences. The MBTI is a widely used and useful instrument when trying to understand the role of individual differences in the learning process. MBTI (www .humanmetrics.com/cgiwin/JTypes2.asp) scores indicate one's preference on each of following four dimensions:

■ Extroversion (E) or Introversion (I)
■ Sensing (S) or Intuition (I)

- Thinking (T) or Feeling (F)
- Judging (J) or Perceiving (P)

Each Myers Briggs type infers a different preference for learning.

TABLE 2.1   Examples of Learning Strategies Based on Multiple Intelligences

MULTIPLE INTELLIGENCE	CHARACTERISTICS OF LEARNERS	LEARNING STRATEGIES
Visual/spatial intelligence	Tend to think in pictures	Charts, maps, visuals, metaphors, graphs, diagrams
Verbal/linguistic intelligence	Learn by speaking and listening	Stories, notes, reading, memorizing, analyzing case studies, text
Logical/mathematical intelligence	Use reason and logic, and ask "why?"	Spreadsheets, experiments, interviewing, classifying and organizing, developing theories, solving problems
Bodily/kinesthetic intelligence	Have the ability to control body movements and handle physical objects. Interact with the space around them	Hands-on manipulation, watching videos or presentations, simulations, games, videoconferencing, creating something with hands
Musical/rhythmical intelligence	Appreciates and produces music with sounds, rhythms, and patterns	Compose songs, tones, and sound effects
Interpersonal intelligence	Have an advanced ability to relate to and understand the feelings of others.	Telling stories about how other people feel, learning teams, small group discussion, role playing, analyzing case studies, and consensus- or agreement-building exercises
Intrapersonal intelligence	Exhibit a strong sense of self and the ability to understand and share inner thoughts and feelings	Surveys, role-playing, discussion
Naturalist intelligence	Have an appreciation for and an understanding of the world around them	Like the outdoors and animals, exploration, investigation, field trips, tours

THEORIES IN EDUCATION

Distance-based learning is a complex event that cannot be explained with a single learning theory, according to Johnson and Aragon (2003). Instead, quality-learning environments should be based on instructional principles that are derived from multiple learning theories. Theories about learning are mostly derived from psychology and education. While psychology describes how people act, educational theory describes how people learn and come to make sense of the world around them. This section presents educational theories and strategies to better understand learning and to effectively prepare educational programs.

Behavioral Theory

Behaviorism is based upon traditional beliefs about how we learn and is one of the most influential theories in the fields of education and psychology. Ivan Pavlov (1849–1936) conducted experiments in Russia with dogs. He rang a bell and then gave the dogs food. He repeated the ringing of the bell and the giving of food over and over until the dogs began to salivate in anticipation of food when the bell rang. This stimulus response behavior is called classical conditioning. Edward Thorndike (1874–1949) applied behaviorism to education at Columbia University in New York. He postulated that learning was the resultant connection between a stimulus and a response. B. F. Skinner (1904–1990) continued work with stimulus response but focused on studying voluntary responses. He rewarded responses that were desirable and punished or ignored undesirable responses. His work is called operant conditioning. His theory, like those of Pavlov and Thorndike, was based on behavioral change while mental processes were ignored. Behavioral change is what is observed—that is, what one says or does, or how one behaves. If a behavior is observed, it is the response to a stimulus. A stimulus is defined as an object in the environment that poses a physiologic threat. A response is anything that one does in response to a stimulus. It could be as simple as a turn of the head, a twitch, or saying, "I am sorry," or as complex as designing a building or writing a book. Behaviorism was popular until the 1950s, but it began to lose supporters because the theory explained learning from only a behavioral perspective and is therefore limited in scope. The psychological theory of behaviorism is used as an educational theory when the learning experience is based on a stimulus and a response, and by rewarding behavior that will meet the educational goal and ignoring (or correcting) behavior that is not goal directed. In behavioral theory, large tasks are broken down into smaller tasks, and each task is learned in successive order. The process is called successive approximations. Behaviorist-based instructional practice is usually teacher centered and designed around the instructor presenting information and the students passively receiving that information and presenting the knowledge they acquired back to the instructor for assessment. Traditional learning labs are an example of behaviorist theory. In this environment a student may be learning the correct procedure for a dry, sterile dressing. Using behavioral practices, the instruction is focused on taking the entire procedure and breaking it down into steps, learners master the first step then move to successive steps until they master every step to complete the procedure. The first steps would be to verify the order, then gather equipment, and then prepare the client, set up the area for a sterile field, and so forth. By learning a segment at a time and doing each segment correctly, the student will be able to successfully complete the dry sterile dressing procedure by putting the learned steps together.

Constructivist Theory

While some educators believe that although the teacher imparts information it does not necessarily mean that the student will learn. Constructivist educators believe that learning occurs when the learner synthesizes and makes sense of new information and connects the new information to existing understandings or schema. Thinking inspires learning. Thinking is stimulated through activities. It is the teacher who provides the content and the activities that initiate and motivate the learners to involve themselves in the activities and thus to think. Thinking helps learners transform information to their context or to a context personal to them and thus see ways to use the information in their lives. Learning becomes the responsibility of the learner; instruction is student-centered rather than teacher-centered. Jonassen, Peck, Wilson, and Pfeiffer (1998) contrast traditional learning and constructivism. In traditional learning, knowledge is transmitted and is external to the learner, whereas in constructivist learning, knowledge is constructed by the learner's action, experience, and perceptions. In traditional learning methods, learning is the transfer of knowledge from the teacher to the student with an emphasis on the outcome. Constructivist learning focuses on interpreting the world and constructing meaning. Learning is active and reflective, which means that there is doing, then reflecting about the doing, and then rethinking about the doing. Action and reflection enable the student to integrate new knowledge with existing knowledge and experiences so that complex mental models can form. Integrating old and the new learning allows the student to look at the world from a unique perspective. Learning is authentic and resembles real-life experiences.

Constructivist learning is process oriented with an emphasis on collaboration and conversation among learners and teachers. In the traditional classroom, instruction is the imparting of information from the top down using a deductive thinking process. Learning is competitive and is controlled by the instructor. In the constructivist approach instruction is inductive, from the bottom up. Learning opportunities are diverse and increase in complexity. The instructor is a model and a coach who encourages exploration of ideas, and learning is learner centered and learner generated. Constructivism assumes that learning is personal and that the student brings past knowledge and experience to the learning situation. Constructivism is the process of bringing new knowledge to past experiences to construct a new reality and to make sense and meaning out of the world. How do students construct their own reality? It is through engaging in an active learning process. Active learning is an approach that engages the student in thinking and rethinking, thus creating new ideas. Students interact with the environment (content, faculty, activities, and peers). Active learning, according to Dodge (n.d.), involves the process of providing students with situations that require them to read, speak, listen, think, and write. Although lectures may be well written and well delivered, they often pass from the ear to the hand, leaving the mind untouched. The active learning process places responsibility on the learners themselves and lends itself to a wider range of learning styles.

Active learning on the web involves taking a critical look at the resources that already exist and incorporating them into the learning environment. Examples might include web quests, blogs, or wikis that would require learners to research information, and then return to the online class environment to further collaborate and expand on their research findings. Learning environments must be rich with strategies and resources so the student can construct meaning from content, faculty, activities, and peers. Technology can provide the richness that constructivist learning environments require to guide knowledge construction. Construction of knowledge is the result of social interaction.

Social Interaction

Social interaction has long been thought to increase collaboration and therefore result in increased learning. Jung, Choi, Lim, and Leem (2002) studied interactions in groups and learning outcomes and concluded that adult learners who engaged in social interaction with their instructors and collaborative interaction with peers scored higher on outcome measures of learning than adult learners who did not engage in social and collaborative interaction. This interaction continues to be recognized as one of the most important components of learning experiences both in conventional education and distance education (Bacalarski, n.d.). Research findings suggest that learning in groups improves students' achievement of learning objectives. Vygotsky (1978) believed that cognitive development and learning are dependent on social interaction. The major theme of this theoretical framework is that social interaction plays a fundamental role in the process of learning. A second aspect of Vygotsky's theory is the idea that the potential for cognitive development is limited to a certain "time span," which he refers to as the zone of proximal development (ZPD). It is during this time that consciousness is raised and a range of skills can be developed with adult guidance or peer collaboration. Vygotsky's methods of analysis and conclusions about the development of human thought and language are still considered accurate today and can be applied to the study of computer-mediated communication.

Problem-Based Learning

Problem-based learning (PBL) is an instructional method that involves the presentation of a clinical problem as a teaching strategy (Ridley, 2007). Donner and Bickley (1993) described PBL as a form of education that allows for information to be mastered in the same context in which it is used. PBL, because of its ability to provide for an authentic problem as the stimulus for learning, fulfills the requirements of a cognitive apprenticeship as described by Brown, Collins, and Duguid (1989).

PBL has the characteristics of a constructivist, student-centered learning environment as advocated by Jonassen (2000). In this environment learners are provided with a question, issue, case, project, or problem that they attempt to solve. This student-centered approach replaces lectures with active learning and holds students responsible for their development of knowledge. In addition, this environment allows the learners to pursue learning at their own pace and explore increasingly complex levels of content to meet their learning needs. Within PBL, students learn content and apply it in an authentic situation to answer the question or solve the problem. PBL, because if its ability to elicit problem solving and critical analysis, endeavors to bridge the gap between theoretical knowledge and practical application. Medical schools in the United States began utilizing PBL in the 1970s and since then it has become commonplace. More recently, PBL has been incorporated as a teaching method in the education of other health professionals including nurses, physical therapists, and public health professionals.

The PBL process is structured in four specific phases. Phase one involves students reasoning through the problem and identifying their learning needs in groups. The next phase consists of learners engaging in self-directed learning as they explore the topic. In phase three, the group process takes over with each learner applying the results of individual research to the problem. Finally the fourth phase involves the summary of the information gathered and utilization of this information in problem solving (Neville, 2009).

Learners are assisted in their pursuit of knowledge by an instructor who is more expert in the area than the learners. In line with constructivist approaches to learning, the instructor facilitates but does not direct or dictate learning. Learning is accomplished independently by the learners, but is greatly supported by the participation of the instructor who provides guidance in the discovery process. The learners also benefit from the pre-existing knowledge and research shared by other group members in pursuit of problem resolution. Woltering, Herrler, Spitzer, and Spreckelsen (2009) found that medical students using online PBL had an increased motivation for learning and higher satisfaction with their learning gains over students in the traditional PBL environment. The online support of the PBL process had benefits for the students and resulted in improved cooperation. King et al. (2010) studied online PBL in an interprofessional health sciences course and found that the online learning environment facilitated small group collaborative interactions. Conducting PBL online could be advantageous to increasing discipline-specific skills, team skills, and fluency with information technology. The online environment allows students to utilize a variety of resources beyond traditional textbooks to pursue self-directed learning, an essential feature of PBL as a constructivist method of instruction. Hill, Wiley, Nelson, and Han (2004) argued that "learning with" Internet resources allowed students to actively construct something unique as they used the Internet for information gathering. Internet resources utilized in this manner become "cognitive tools" that enhanced human thinking, problem solving, and learning. Moreover, students preferred the ability to gather information at their own pace to construct solutions to problems. The variety of online resources available also helps support individual learning styles.

PBL has the ability to improve students' critical-thinking skills and motivation for learning, and to enhance student autonomy and self-direction. Furthermore, PBL increases students' ability to apply their learning to practice and enables them to use a variety of resources to pursue learning. These features of PBL can enable students to become more effective practitioners and lifelong learners.

TECHNOLOGY AND LEARNING

Technology has traditionally been used for the purpose of conveying information to students. Howland, Jonassen, and Marra (2011) argue that technology does more than that—technology can be used to support the student's creation of meaning out of learning. Technology can foster learning and thinking because it is a vehicle for exploring; allows for access to information; supports learning by doing through case studies and simulations; and supports interaction.

PULLING IT ALL TOGETHER FOR GOOD PEDAGOGY

So, how can we bring developmental theory, learning style, learning theory, and technology together to create effective learning environments? Undergraduate nursing education traditionally includes faculty-developed behavioral objectives and instructional materials along with evaluation that focuses on the attainment of these objectives. This faculty-centered approach is an example of behaviorism.

Here is the dilemma: Behaviorism is teacher centered, and online learning should be student centered. Nursing education and training tends toward behaviorism, and the literature supports constructivism as the online approach to effective learning. If teacher-centered objectives and evaluation of outcomes are necessities, techniques can be used to make the behaviorist favor constructivist components and thereby become more student centered. One technique is to include assessments of student learning styles and structured learning experiences to accommodate those learning styles. Once a student's learning style is assessed, instructors should develop a prescriptive plan for each student to guide his or her learning. Objectives can be written in a behavioral format, but students can provide or work with real-life case studies to analyze and thus meet objectives. When a combination of behaviorist and constructivist approaches is used, the learning is called a "guided constructivist learning model."

If guided constructivism were the theory used to design online learning environments, objectives would be learning centered and would guide the learning experience. Emphasis would be placed on the process of knowledge construction rather than on the outcomes of learning. Content would be presented to accommodate various learning styles and developmental levels, and an emphasis would be placed on active learning through questions, case studies, and projects that would help the student develop mental models and test reality. These approaches allow the student to apply basic information to real-world practice. Experimenting with your student population, instructional beliefs, and varied practices will help you to find the best ways to design effective online instruction.

REFERENCES

Bacalarski, M. (n.d.). Vygotski's developmental theories and the adulthood of computer mediated communication: A comparison and an illumination. Retrieved from http://psych.hanover.edu/vygotsky/bacalar.html

Brown, J., Collins, A., & Duguid, P. (1989). Situated cognition and the culture of learning. *Educational Researcher, 18*(1), 32–42. Retrieved from http://www .aera.net/publications/?id=317

Dodge, B. (n.d.). Active learning on the web. Retrieved from http://edweb.sdsu.edu/people/bdodge/Active/ActiveLearning.html

Donner, R., & Bickley, H. (1993). Problem-based learning in American medical education: An overview. *Bulletin of the Medical Library Association, 81*(3), 294–298. Retrieved from http://www.ncbi.nlm.nih.gov/pmc/articles/PMC225793

Educational Broadcasting Company. (2004). Concept to classroom: Tapping into multiple intelligences. Retrieved from http://www.thirteen.org/edonline/concept2class/mi/index.html

Hill, J., Wiley, D., Nelson, L. M., & Han, S. (2004). Exploring research on internet-based learning: From infrastructure to interactions. In D. Jonassen (Ed.), *Handbook of Research on Educational Communications and Technology* (pp. 433–459). Mahwah, NJ: Lawrence Erlbaum Associates, Inc. Retrieved from http://www.questia.com/PM.qst?a=o&d=10487577

Howland, J., Jonassen, D., & Marra, R. M. (2011). *Meaningful learning with technology.* (4th ed). Columbus, OH: Merrill/Prentice Hall.

Johnson, S., & Aragon, S. (2003). An instructional strategy framework for online learning environments. *New Directions for Adult and Continuing Education, 100,* 31–43.

Jonassen, D. (2000). *Computers as mindtools in schools: Engaging critical thinking.* Columbus, OH: Merrill/Prentice Hall.

Jonassen, D. (2000). Revisiting activity theory as a framework for designing student-centered learning environments. In D. Jonassen & S. M. Land (Eds.), *Theoretical foundations of learning environments* (pp. 89–122). Mahwah, NJ: Lawrence Erlbaum Associates, Inc.

Jonassen, D. H., Peck, K. L., Wilson, B. G., & Pfeiffer, W. S. (1998). *Learning with technology: A constructivist perspective.* Upper Saddle River, NJ: Prentice Hall.

Jung, I., Choi, S., Lim, C., & Leem, J. (2002). Effects of different types of interaction on learning achievement, satisfaction and participation in web-based instruction. *Innovations in Education and Teaching International, 39*(2), 153–162.

Knowles, M. (1970). *The modern practice of adult education: Andragogy versus pedagogy.* New York: The Association Press.

Meacham, M. (2003). Using multiple intelligence theory in the virtual classroom. Retrieved from http://www.learningcircuits.org/2003/jun2003/elearn.html

Neville, A. J. (2009). Problem-based learning and medical education forty years on: A review of its effects on knowledge and clinical performance. *Medical Principles and Practice. 18*(1):1–9.

Pelz, B. (2004). (My) three principles of effective online pedagogy. *Journal of Asynchronous Learning Networks, 8*(3).

Ridley, R. (2007). Interactive teaching: A concept analysis. *Journal of Nursing Education*, 46(5), 203–209. Retrieved from http://www.journalofnursing education.com

Vygotsky, L. (1978). *Mind in society: The development of higher psychological processes*. Cambridge, MA: Harvard University Press.

Woltering, V., Herrler, A., Spitzer, K., & Spreckelsen, C. (2009). Blended learning positively affects students' satisfaction and the role of the tutor in the problem-based learning process: Results of a mixed-method evaluation. *Advances in Health Science Education*, 14, 725–738. doi:10.1007/s10459-009-9154-6

Infrastructure Considerations for Online Learning: Student Faculty and Technical Support

CHERYL A. FISHER

The growth in broadband, mobile technology, and adaptive multimedia is both shifting and enhancing the experiences for distance learners. The available combinations of innovative pedagogic strategies have provided and encouraged novel learning technologies (Wade & Ashman, 2007). However, the challenge remains to provide stimulating learning environments supported by technology.

The technical infrastructure necessary to support distance learning is critical when planning distance programs and includes a conglomeration of policies, services, and resources designated to support distance learning efforts. Although distance learning is becoming more and more mainstream, not all academic institutions have an infrastructure in place to support the effort. Building infrastructure is dependent on institutional and technological resources, student support services, and faculty support. This chapter will address major factors and trends that are impacting academic institutions and distance education programs within the broad scope of the supporting infrastructure.

INSTITUTIONAL CONSIDERATIONS

Often, the institution's mission statement and strategic plan are good places to start looking for evidence of technology support for online learning. Often these documents will serve as the drivers for a technical infrastructure that will support distance learning programs.

For example, Pennsylvania State University (www.psu.edu/), a longstanding leader in distance education, uses guiding principles for infrastructure to support distance education. These are based on policy, a dynamic programmatic mission, student and faculty support, and the need for policy change to support distance education efforts. Pennsylvania State University maintains that distance education is best recognized as an integrated part of the college-wide strategic goals and not as a separate activity.

When comparing strategic plans among similar large universities, several commonalities can be noted. These common elements include:

- An inclusive planning process with broad-based constituency involvement
- A clear statement of the institution's mission and its aspirations for its current planning period
- Comprehensive goals directly traceable to attainment of these aspirations and advancement of the institution's mission
- Clearly defined outcomes to assess the plan's success against nationally accepted measures

A technical infrastructure is not directly mentioned in the common elements; however, this cannot be obtained without the ability to reach a broad-based constituency. To do this successfully, the institution should have a web presence and outcome measures that utilize strong database management and networking capability.

Within nursing, the American Association of Colleges of Nursing (AACN, 2013) identifies factors that need to be addressed by nurses and other leaders in education and health care institutions, as well as external funders and policy makers, in order to take full advantage of the benefits of technology-supported education. These factors include:

- Superior distance education programs require substantial institutional financial investment in equipment, infrastructure, and faculty development.
- Local, regional, and national planning for multisite communications needs to consider coordination of services, compatibility and progressive upgrading of hardware, as well as policies that lower transmission costs within and across state lines.
- The use of distance technology, and web-based media in particular, has raised questions regarding intellectual property and copyrights, privacy of educational dialogue, and other related legal and ethical issues that require continued clarification.
- Technology-mediated teaching strategies can dramatically change the way teaching and learning occur, challenging the traditional relationship of students to academic institutions. These strategies may change conventional thinking about how the quality of educational programs is assessed and what is required to support student learning (e.g., library access, counseling services, computing, tuition, and financial aid).
- Nursing schools that use distance education technology have an advantage in recruiting students, and nursing schools are competing for students in their distance programs.

With supporting documents and other structural supports in place, an institution can better assess and plan where to focus resources and efforts necessary for a successful online program infrastructure. A review of institutional strategic plans conducted by Tallent Runnels, Thomas, Lan, Cooper, Ahern, Shaw, and Liu (2006) revealed that few universities have policies, guidelines, or technical support for faculty members or students. However, since the time of Tallent Runnels et al.'s review, most academic settings have come to realize the importance of these services and support structures for stakeholders, and samples can be easily found on their websites. For example, Indiana University School of Nursing (nursing.iupui.edu/continuing/resources.shtml) has a web page for helping students new to online learning get started with simple instructions. The University of Illinois (www.online.uillinois.edu/resources/supporttraining.asp) has faculty and student support services, resources, and training available to ensure success.

The American Distance Education Consortium (ADEC, 2012) is a nonprofit, distance education consortium composed of approximately

65 state universities and land-grant colleges. The consortium was developed to promote the creation and provision of high quality, economical distance education programs and services to diverse audiences by the land grant community of colleges and universities, through the most appropriate information technologies available.

As a collaborative partner with Alfred P. Sloan Foundation, National Association of State Universities and Land Grant Colleges (NASULGC), and several government agencies (National Science Foundation, U.S. Department of Agriculture, National Agriculture Library, and others), ADEC sets forth goals that specify support to empower visionary thinking about education and technology. These goals are centered on collaboration of people, environments, hardware and connectivity, and software-driven tools that encourage and enhance teaching and learning specifically to engage people in the learning environment. These initiatives address key issues, including global reach, research, and workforce development, all of which are critical elements for successful program development and expansion.

The consortium utilizes the best subject matter experts and information resources to share knowledge and content with learners. ADEC programming is offered virtually as well as locally, regionally, nationally, and internationally, and is characterized by the following guiding principles:

- Design for active and effective learning
- Support the needs of learners
- Develop and maintain the technological and human infrastructure
- Sustain administrative and organizational commitment

INFORMATION TECHNOLOGY

When addressing technological issues for distance learning, ADEC recommends that institutions establish appropriate technical requirements. This requires that compatibility needs be met, that technology at origination and reception sites ensure quality, that learners and facilitators be supported in their use of these technologies, and that collaboration efforts be explored. It is becoming increasingly common to find institutional settings seeking external collaboration opportunities in order to share resources to meet these requirements.

Collaboration, consortia, and other alliances allow campuses to contribute content and resources to specific courses or areas of study in order to make most efficient use of time and money. The Connecticut Distance Learning Consortium (2013) is one example in which a collaborative e-tutoring program has been created to meet the online needs of participating 2-year and 4-year public and private institutions of higher education. This interinstitutional program operates via a collaborative process that facilitates the sharing of tutors, workshops, resources, and research opportunities by all members for a low cost. In addition, the collaboration among schools enables ongoing development of effective best practices protocols, as well as the design and delivery of an online tutoring platform that enables both synchronous and asynchronous tutoring opportunities. Other services available to members include learning management hosting, instructional design, web integration, technical support, and strategic consulting.

The Western Interstate Commission for Higher Education (WICHE, 2013) was created in the 1950s by the Western states to promote resource sharing, collaboration, and cooperative planning among their higher education systems. This collaboration seeks to improve access to higher education through the use of technology and to ensure student success. Now a system with 15 states, members share information, technical expertise, services, and equipment related to distance learning.

Similarly, Iowa Communications Network (ICN, 2013), invests in educational telecommunications and technology to support two-way interactive video conferencing in support of distance learning. The ICN is the country's premier fiber optic network, committed to continued enhancement of distance learning. It provides Iowans with convenient access to educational resources and support. The network makes it possible for remote and physically separated Iowans to interact in an efficient and cost-effective manner, utilizing partnerships with education, medicine, and government agencies. In 2012, the ICN Annual Report stated that data services and bandwidth tripled over previous years and that 85% of the Internet services are being used for educational purposes.

STUDENT SUPPORT SERVICES

Online distance learners require multiple layers of support. Support services are critical to the success for the course and for the retention of online distance learners (Smith & Curry, 2005). These services include administrative support, technical support, mentor support, and other services.

Administrative support is often required in several forms, including admissions, finance, registration, advising, and extension or deferral requests. It is imperative that student support be available and user friendly and that the responsible administrative personnel be adequately trained in providing these services. Often administrative support is offered in the form of a help desk or online help site with email addresses, phone numbers, and frequently asked questions (FAQs) for distance learning students. An example of this type of site can be found on the Clemson University website (http://www.clemson .edu/ccit/learning_tech/distance_ed/index.html).

Counseling services need to be available to distance learning students and can be provided via synchronous or asynchronous means (live chat or email) or by telephone. Student counseling centers often educate through informational pamphlets on various topics. The commercially available options are limited to specialized topics relevant to students. A counseling center can produce its own pamphlets, however, but that would be costly and time consuming. Most universities now provide counseling service information via the web and provide links for counseling topics and resources. However, human resources remain essential to ensure that all necessary information is appropriate and up to date.

The National Academic Advising Association Technology in Advising Commission (NACADA, 2013) out of Kansas State University suggests distance learning students should have the same advising and counseling resources available to them that on campus students have. These include workshops or training in the use of distance education technologies as required for students enrolled in courses or programs; access to the appropriate learning resources as required of distance learning students (i.e., basic skills, course tutorials, disability support, library services, and so forth); accurate information on the assumptions about the technical competence and skill level required; accurate and timely information; and an internal distance learner network that connects all processes required of the distance learners and provides them with one point of contact for the services.

The NACADA website (http://www.nacada.ksu.edu) also lists academic advising resources available on the Internet, including topics ranging from career counseling to study skills, as well as multiple listing of academic advising web page links to universities across the country. The core values described by NACADA reflect the fact that advisement is a personal process and establishes a relationship between the students and their advisors. Further, when done correctly, advisement is not just between the student and the advisor, but involves a team effort that includes the student support services of the institution, the student, and the advisor. Carnevale (2000) identified guidelines for developing an advising site for students based on WICHE and NACADA. This advising site should include the following elements:

1. *A clear and concise explanation of core curriculum (or general education) requirements.* Advisement usually involves a comprehensive explanation of curriculum requirements and a review of what a student has left to complete. Making this information available online will free up some time, will give students greater control and responsibility for the advisement process, and will provide essential information for students trying to determine course selection if they are unable to meet with an advisor.

2. *An FAQ section.* Every advisor spends a portion of the day repeating answers to the same questions. Putting answers to FAQs online saves time for staff and gives students access to answers as needed.

3. *Informational pages for special populations and self-help assistance.* While there are certain common needs among students, there are segments of the population with unique concerns. Freshmen, students without declared majors, students on academic probation, and commuters are examples of groups with additional need for support. Examples of information to include for advisement are career or major information, study skills-building worksheets, an explanation of the academic standing policy, information on how to get computer access and technical support, and parking information should onsite visits be necessary.

4. *Links to related university sites.* Holistic advisement involves supporting a student both academically and personally. Links to campus services such as student activity calendars, campus organization pages, career services, academic lab locations and hours, and intramural offerings are necessary to ensure all needs are being met.

5. *One-on-one access to advisors.* To generate a more personal environment and provide opportunities for interaction, advisors are experimenting with various forms of electronic communications. This is the most critical element in a comprehensive advising website. If advising were simply a matter of giving students a standardized package of information, there would be no reason to have advisors. Access to a qualified advisor can be achieved through the use of live chat, listservs, and emails, to mention a few of the most common methods.

WICHE (2001) evaluated online student support offerings at 15 colleges and universities and selected what they identified as best practices for integrating technology into student support services. The services evaluated a range from advisement and personal counseling to registration and financial aid. In 2003, WICHE went on to develop a "cheat sheet" to help organizations with general directions for developing online student services. These steps include:

1. Form a vision team and develop your campus's vision for student services online.
2. Determine the initial focus of student services and assemble a project design and development team.
3. Create a glossary of terms for student services and define the scope, budget, and timeline.
4. Write scenarios and record ARIs (assumptions, requirements, and issues).
5. Identify affected policies and take steps to address them.
6. Buy, build, or partner in the development of a technology solution to support plans for new service(s).
7. Test the new service with a pilot group of students.
8. Form an implementation team and develop an implementation plan.
9. Deploy your new service(s), gaining a yield of integrated information technology (IT) systems, simple procedures, and online services.
10. Keep your institution happy with well-served students, faculty, staff, and others by upgrading the service(s) on an ongoing basis to maintain state-of-the-art services.

INFORMATION FOR PROSPECTIVE STUDENTS

The services recommended should begin with the first encounter that students are likely to have with a university when looking for an online course or program. The university home page should include information for students to help them decide if this is the right place for them. There should be clear and highly visible information about online programs with direct links to more in-depth information. A short self-assessment quiz can help students determine if they are ready for online learning. An example of this self-assessment quiz can be found on the website of Old Dominion University (clt.odu .edu/oso/index.php?src=pe_isdlforme). Such questions can help students determine how distance education will fit their individual needs and will reinforce the requirements of commitment and independent work in online environments. This site also helps students to assess their computer requirements and their computer literacy in order to determine if they will be a successful online student and if this is the best option for them.

Although these tools do not provide assurance of success, they help students identify technical skills and learning styles that will help them be successful online learners. A hardware and software assessment should be provided to students so they can determine the specifications necessary to participate in a course. A list of hardware, software, Internet service provider requirements, email, and browser requirements should be specified with definitions of terms included. An FAQ page is also often helpful, along with contact information such as email addresses or phone numbers for students to get additional information.

ADMISSIONS

The admissions process should be clearly delineated with specific steps for each part of the process. Admission requirements should be identified with program-specific criteria to help students decide if they, in fact, want to apply. Methods for obtaining and submitting an application, deadlines, application tracking, and multiple payment methods are also recommended.

As previously mentioned, another early step in the process that students should consider is a computer self-assessment. Many universities offering online education have these assessments available on the home page of their websites. These assessments usually cover basic skills in Windows® and email, and provide hardware and software requirements.

ADVISING

NACADA states that providers of distance education programs must offer a minimum set of core services that assist distance learners in identifying and achieving their education goals. To facilitate this goal attainment, the following standards have been developed to address many categories as identified by the Academic Advising Council for the Advancement of Standards (CAS). These standards have been divided into three main categories: institutional, faculty advisor standards, and student standards. NACADA suggests the following standards for faculty advisors:

- A distance education program must provide for appropriate, real-time or delayed interaction among faculty, advisors, and students.
- The program must provide faculty and advisor with support to assist students in making informed choices about career and academic goals, self-assessment, decision making, and evaluation of academic career options.
- The program must provide faculty and advisor with the support to orient students to the distance learning environment.
- The institution must provide an environment in which faculty and advisors can work toward achieving competencies needed to be an advisor of distance learners.

Although advising is critical for all students, it is even more essential that distance students feel they have a connection to someone at the institution. As these guidelines recommend, if students are to be successful, they need more than just quality courses online.

Content and learning support are also important to distance learning programs and may require services from tutors, writing centers, or campus libraries. The Western Cooperative for Telecommunications Education (2008) created a guide for developing distance student services. These guidelines discuss tips for developing these services, as well as a discussion on the range of services that should be included and guidelines for best practices in delivering these services online. Although universities have increasingly recognized the value and need to provide online courses and programs, they often need help envisioning what services to provide and how to design them. The services addressed in this guide for students were determined to be "good practices" based on interactive web services or for-profit companies that market software to support student needs. The student support services identified include:

- Information for prospective students
- Admissions
- Financial aid
- Registration
- Orientation services
- Academic advising
- Technical support
- Career services
- Library services
- Services for students with disabilities
- Personal counseling
- Instructional support and counseling
- Bookstore
- Services to promote a sense of community

Financial Aid

Financial aid is a critical factor for students in the educational choices that they make. The issue of financial aid has an impact on course load, institutional choice, and whether the student can pursue higher education. Because of its importance, students should be able to easily access all financial aid information and forms directly from the web. The information should include general information about financial aid, types of aid, details of cost, and the application process. The institution's financial aid policies should be disclosed for students in addition to federal school codes for the federal financial aid application. Dates, deadlines for application, and links to related sites are also important information sources and include general information for students.

Registration

Registration for online students is probably one of the most important online services that must be available and user friendly. This service will be used when students are registering for a program and each time they register for a course. Good practice recommendations include a full description of the registration process, identification of all registration method options available, relevant policies, an online scheduler, and online registration forms with clear instructions.

Software for online student registration is now readily available and easier to use, with increasing ability to meet student and higher education demands. Available are features such as student registration, database course management, credit card payment capability, and custom report writing, just to mention a few. Additional features include financial aid application capability, records and registration, and the billing system. PeopleSoft, Zen grade Corp, e Class Trak, and Aceware are some examples of software available for course management, which are actually suites of products designed to meet the needs of higher educational institutions including institutional resources, student information, financial information, and human resources, among others. Various components can be used for faculty, students, advisors, and employees. These web-based systems have the ability to be accessed anytime and anywhere in response to calls for flexibility and easy access to support services.

Library Services

The Association of College and Research Libraries (ACRL, 2011) calls for resources and services in institutions of higher education to meet the needs of faculty, students, and academic support personnel, regardless of where they are located. Special funding, proactive planning, and promotion are necessary to deliver equivalent library services to achieve equivalent results in teaching and learning, and generally to maintain quality in distance learning programs.

Reasons given for expanding the ACRL guidelines for distance learners have initiated from the fact that nontraditional study is rapidly becoming a major element in higher education, with an increase in the diversity of educational opportunities, an increase in the number of unique environments where educational opportunities are offered, an increased recognition for the need for library services, and the requirement for services at locations other than main campuses (ACLR, 2008). Often it is the classroom that may have greater needs for library services. With the increase in technological innovation in the transmittal of information, a shift has been created toward an all-electronic university.

The library services recommended should be designed to effectively provide a wide range of information services and to be responsive to user needs. According to the ACRL, the following services, though not all inclusive, are essential:

1. Reference assistance
2. Computer-based bibliographic and informational services
3. Reliable, rapid, and secure access to institutional and other networks, including the Internet
4. A program of library user instruction designed to instill independent and effective information literacy skills while specifically meeting the learner support needs of the distance learning community
5. Assistance with and instruction in the use of nonprint media and equipment
6. Reciprocal or contractual borrowing or interlibrary loan services using the broadest application of fair use of copyrighted materials
7. Prompt document delivery such as a courier system or electronic transmission
8. Access to reserve materials in accordance with copyright fair use policies
9. Adequate service hours for optimum access by users and consultative services
10. Promotion of library services to the distance learning community, including documented and updated policies, regulations, and procedures for systematic development and management of information resources.

As demand for electronic delivery of these services increases, demand for additional texts, journals, and other resources have also increased. The student website should include general information, services, tools, and technical help for students and faculty.

Faculty Support and Workload

Faculty support is another major consideration that institutions need to consider when developing distance programs. The time, knowledge, and skills that are required to design, develop, and teach online cannot be taken for granted or assumed by administrators to be basic faculty skills. Many institutions now are employing instructional designers and onsite technical support for course development since the demand has dramatically increased over the past several years.

Faculty training for distance education has not traditionally been addressed by university settings. It is now becoming more widely recognized that teaching online is different from teaching in the classroom. As the value and complexity of this endeavor is realized, more institutions are investing time and resources into faculty training. The Indiana Higher Education Telecommunication System (IHETS, 2013) recommends that institutions engaged in the delivery of distance learning provide appropriate training experiences for their faculty. IHETS suggests that faculty be exposed to various pedagogical strategies that are well suited to the distance learning environment, and that exposure to inservices, workshops, and interactions with experienced peers be provided. Often this training is offered online.

IHETS identified the following principles and subprinciples relevant to faculty development. The main principle is that it is important for faculty who are engaged in the delivery of distance learning courses to take advantage of appropriate professional developmental experiences. The subprinciples include:

1. Faculty will seek out and participate in opportunities that expose them to various pedagogical strategies that are well suited to the distance learning environment. This exposure could come from participation in inservices and workshops.
2. Faculty will seek out opportunities for collaborations and other interactions with faculty that have had success in the distance learning environment. Those faculty members who have had success in distance learning should take a mentorship role with those who are seeking assistance.
3. Faculty will participate in the evaluation and selection of the software products that are going to be used for course development. Faculty should seek out and participate in ongoing training and technical support for various distance learning development and delivery tools.

4. Faculty will understand the implications of teaching via distance, for example, the unique challenges presented by the various technologies.
5. Faculty will understand and observe the institution's policies regarding intellectual property and copyright.

These principles put the responsibility for course design and online facilitation on the faculty teaching the course. Ideally, faculty support for course development should include technical support, assurance of basic technical skills required to offer online courses, and available resources for support. Courses are now available online to learn the basic principles of teaching online. For example, Maryland Online has a course available that was designed and developed by expert faculty from six different institutions. The Certificate for Online Adjunct Teaching (COAT, 2013) course is an online training course designed for instructors who are interested in learning how to teach online. Originally designed for adjunct instructors, full-time instructors, instructional designers, and administrators also find the course to be valuable. This course can be found at marylandonline.org/coat/.

Faculty workload is a key factor that must be considered and defined. "Faculty workload" is defined as how much a faculty member teaches and how much of his or her work time is taken up with research, administration, and other duties. IHETS (2013) recommends a system of faculty incentives and rewards be developed cooperatively by faculty and the administration that encourages effort and recognizes achievement associated with the development and delivery of distance learning courses. Additional recommendations include a mechanism for determining whether distance learning course development and delivery will be included as part of a faculty member's workload or assigned on an overload basis. The evaluation process according to IHETS should be in accordance with institutional policy for teaching face-to-face courses.

Intellectual property and copyright law issues arise around who owns an electronic course or source materials once it is created. Does it belong to the institution, faculty member, or both? Historically, universities have given copyrights to faculty, allowing them to do as they wish with materials falling under copyright. However, when a faculty member develops a new invention or process, most campuses defined this creative contribution under their patent policies, because the institution had to commit a significant set of resources, and thus there was a sharing of any benefits derived from this intellectual property. Similarly, institutions could claim that when a course is developed using the university's software and university resources, significant institutional resources have been invested, thereby creating shared property. Thompson (1999) claims in his article, "Intellectual Property Meets Information Technology," that neither copyright nor patent policy is well suited to dealing with distributed learning materials. He argues that campuses have not defined adequate policies or reached a clear understanding of the issues around intellectual property, conflict of interest, and revenue sharing.

Faculty should also be provided with information regarding copyright laws and course content development for distance learning courses. Just because something is on the web does not mean that it is there for the taking. The principle recommended by IHETS for determining copyright law compliance is that content developed for distance learning courses will comply with copyright law. The subprinciples include:

1. The process recommended for determining copyright law compliance is as follows:
   a. Attention will be paid to the rights and privileges regarding transmission of materials as defined in Section 110(2) of the U.S. Copyright Law (http://www.copyright.gov/).
   b. If Section 110(2) does not apply, "fair use," as defined in Section 107, may apply. The nature and amount of the work used, and the purpose and effect of the use will be weighed to determine if fair use applies.
   c. If the planned use of a copyrighted work cannot be addressed by Section 110(2) or Section 107, permission of the content owner may be required.
2. Be aware how to obtain copyright permission. Some institutions may provide assistance in obtaining such permission. A helpful resource for copyright guidance can be found at the National Library of Medicine's website (http://www.nlm.nih.gov/hmd/copyright/copylawguidance.html).

In summary, the importance of institutional commitment from the strategic plan to the home page must be evidenced by faculty support and a complex technological structure. There clearly needs to be a commitment on the part of the institution, the faculty, and the students themselves in order to have a well-supported distance program. When considering recommended guidelines and the multiple systems and resources mentioned throughout this chapter, an organization's strategic plan can help to support the requirements for establishment, maintenance, and growth of a distance program.

REFERENCES

American Association of Colleges of Nursing. (2013). AACN white paper: distance technology in nursing education. Retrieved from http://www.aacn.nche.edu

American Distance Education Consortium (ADEC). (2013). ADEC strategic plan. Retrieved from http://www.adec.edu

Association of College and Research Libraries (ACRL). (2011). Standards and guidelines. Retrieved from http://www.ala.org/acrl/guides/distlrng.html

Carnevale, D. (2000). Commission's web site helps colleges put student services online. *The Chronicle of Higher Education*. Retrieved from http://chronicle.com

Certificate for Online Adjunct Teaching. (2013). Retrieved from http://marylandonline.org/coat/

Connecticut Distance Learning Consortium. (2013). Retrieved from http://www.ctdlc.org

Indiana Higher Education Telecommunication System. (2013). Retrieved from http://www.ihets.org/progserv/networking/itn

Iowa Communications Network. (2013). Retrieved from http://www.icn.state.ia.us

National Academic Advising Association (NACADA). (2013). Retrieved, from http://www.psu.edu/dus/ncta/linkacad.htm

National Association of State Universities of Land Grant Colleges. Retrieved from http://education.stateuniversity.com/pages/2268/National-Association-State-Universities-Land-Grant-Colleges.html

Pennsylvania State University. (2013). Retrieved, from http http://psu.edu

Smith, L., & Curry M. (2005). Teaching tips for authoring online distance learning medical post registration programs. *Medical Teacher, 27*(4), 316–324.

Tallent Runnels, M., Thomas, J., Lan, W., Cooper, L., Ahern, T., Shaw, S., & Liu, X. (2006). Teaching courses online: A review of the research. *Review of Educational Research, 76*(1), 93–135.

Thompson, D. (1999). Intellectual property meets information technology. *Educom Review, 34*(2), 14–21.

Wade, V., & Ashman, H. (2007) Evolving the infrastructure for distance learning. IEEE Computer Society. Retrieved from http://www.bibsonomy.org/bibtex/2812f88dcf9ddff331804fd2793eb9f9e/dblp?layout=simplehtml

Western Interstate Commission for Higher Education. (2013). Retrieved from http://www.wiche.edu

Western Cooperative for Telecommunications Education. (2008). Retrieved from http://www.wcet.info/about

FOUR

Technology and Online Learning

MATTHEW J. RIETSCHEL

Nursing schools utilize technology in all aspects of academic and nonacademic activities. They use learning management systems, content management systems, websites, databases, social media and online library resources to create an online presence for learning to occur. Schools are using web conferencing to conduct online information sessions for prospective students; faculty are using it to hold office hours; and research teams employ web conferencing to assemble members from far distances. Nursing education is using technology to supplement simulations, create virtual environments, engage in online games to mimic real-life situations, utilize electronic health records to simulate patient care, and review patient encounters for additional educational objectives. Nursing schools and licensing bodies are using computer-based assessments to determine if nursing students and registered nurses are prepared to move forward in their coursework and careers. These same practicing and student nurses are using technology to track and log millions of hours of professional development training or clinical hours as required. Finally, the use of Web 2.0 tools has started to find a niche in nursing education, as well as research related to the nursing role. This chapter examines the management systems used in nursing education and the technologies and current trends, programmatic requirements, and student and faculty requirements to be successful in online learning environments.

MANAGEMENT SYSTEMS

There are three main terms that are used when describing management systems; learning, content, and course. The terms are used interchangeably in conversational vernacular when discussing management systems and education because all of the systems are usually accessed via the Internet and content can be loaded either through the same Internet access or by a local network connection. However, the interplay of these terms is not entirely accurate and they draw from different historical contexts. If the terms are examined closely they have very different meanings, although their meanings are usually equated to the context in which they are applied. A learning management system or solution (LMS) is software that has its roots in corporate training and was originally designed for workplace learning environments. A course management system (CMS) is an online system that had its beginnings to partner academic settings. An example of how these systems are used is the delivery of academic courses for credit, professional development of faculty/staff, training for students, and as an online space for organizations and school groups. A content management system (also CMS) is an environment that only stores content for access by other systems or users. This term is not confused with the learning or course management system, as it is a database for the storage of content items for access by other systems or directly by the user. While LMSs offer some content storage options, content management systems offer more general and robust functions for managing content (Piotrowski, 2009). The content management system is not used to deliver education, but rather it is a repository with the ability to upload, manage, and download content artifacts (Catherall, 2008). Another acronym that is commonly used is LCMS, which can represent either learning content management systems or learning course management systems. These terms are used when systems are expanded to include characteristics of multiple systems. These various systems have grown over time and the term learning management system or solution is currently used to define software that can manage, track, and deliver educational programs or courses. Since the terms learning management systems and course management system are used synonymously, this definition can be applied to both terms. The three most popular learning management systems (Dunn, 2012), based on total customers, active users, and online presence, are:

- Moodle: "A software package for producing Internet-based courses and websites. It is a global development project designed to support a social constructionist framework of education" (Moodle, 2013).
- Edmodo: "A free and safe way for students and teachers to connect and collaborate" that "helps connect all learners with the people and resources needed to reach their full potential" (Edmodo, 2013).
- Blackboard: "Blackboard helps clients enrich all aspects of the education experience by engaging and assessing learners, making their daily lives more convenient and secure, and keeping them informed and aware of the most important information" (Blackboard, 2013).

Even though the terms ultimately have different meanings, the meanings are usually equated to the context in which they are applied. Therefore, to understand the capabilities of a specific system, one must look past the term used to describe it and closer at the characteristics of the systems to determine the best solution for their expected use. Since this book is focused on the development of online learning environments, the term used in this chapter to describe the systems will be learning management systems or LMSs.

LMSs have core functionality that allows them to perform the necessary functions for learners, faculty, and administrators. These functions fall into the four categories of communication, administration, productivity tools, and course delivery tools. These four core function areas and the characteristics related to hardware/software and licensing information are all important features to understand in order to choose a system and use it to its full potential. There are websites and services designed to compare the different features; examples are Edutools (2013), which is focused on academic systems, and FindtheBest.com (2013), which compares systems used for corporate learning. Table 4.1 outlines the key features of LMSs that administrators and/or instructors should consult when determining which system will be a good fit for their needs.

The decision on what learning management system to use rarely falls upon faculty. There are some exceptions, usually large institutions

TABLE 4.1   Learning Management System Key Features

Learner Tools	Support Tools	Technical Specifications
Communication Tools • Discussion boards • File storage • Email • Journal/blog • Synchronous chat • Shared workspace (e.g., whiteboard) **Productivity Tools** • Course navigation • Calendar • Progress review • Course content search • Download content • Help **Student Involvement Tools** • Collaborative workspace • Portfolios	**Administration Tools** • Authentication of users • Course authorization • Integration with registration system **Course Delivery Tools** • Assessment management • Feedback tools • Grade book • Course content management • Student progress dashboard **Content Development Tools** • Accessibility compliance • Content management • Course and learning object templates • Customized look and feel • Productivity tools	**Hardware/Software** • Internet browser required • Server requirements for application and stored content (database) **Company Details/Licensing** • Company profile • Costs • Licensing model • Open or proprietary source code • Other options

Source: Adapted from EduTools (2013).

that have multiple systems where faculty will have the opportunity to choose which system they will use to teach a course or training. The ideal method for selecting the LMS for an institution is by a consortium comprised of the informational technology office (technology infrastructure), faculty (needs of the learners and content of the courses), the program directors (curriculum and reporting needs), and the financial group (budget). The process should be a slow one and incorporate all of the LMS feature needs and the requirements of the institution. The faculty and program directors should focus on the learner and support tools as outlined in Table 4.1. The informational technology office and financial group will focus on the technical specifications, which are outlined in Table 4.2.

Along with the learner, support, and technical features to consider, other systems on campus should weigh in on the decision as well. The ideal process for selection of an LMS is to conduct a needs assessment on all of the areas outline previously, decide the most important learner and support tools, and then match the best technical

TABLE 4.2   Comparison of LMS Technical Specifications

Fee Type	• Free • Commercial

Source Code Availability	• Open source
	  – All the files which make up the system are free for modifying, which allows customizing the system in the necessary way
	• Proprietary
	  – Do not provide the source code

Licensing Models	• Per number of registered/enrolled users • Per number of concurrently connected users • Per license validity period • Per number of courses

Installation Type	• Hosted (software as a service)
	  – Installed on the vendor's hardware at their site
	• Own
	  – Installed on the local site or network and provides complete control of all processes

Business Orientation	• eCommerce • Educational institutions • Corporate training • Government structures
Programming Language	• Multiple languages – Important due to impact on technology infrastructure, future programming costs, and other systems desired to integrate
Platform	• Stand-alone solution • Integrated solution

Integration	• Open source
	  – Provides the widest range of integration possibilities
	• Documented application programming interface or API (software development kit or SDK)
	  – Provides the use of one application to be used by another application
	• Integration via bridges
	  – Special plug-ins that allow the integration of different types of applications

Source: Adapted from Joomla (2013).

specifications to meet the academic, infrastructure, and financial needs. While the LMS is the heart of the technology used in teaching an online course, it is not the only technology available to instructors and students. Other technologies can be integrated into the LMS or used as a standalone to supplement the online learning process.

USING TECHNOLOGY IN ONLINE LEARNING

The need to discuss the technologies in categorical terms and not by in-depth exploration of individual, named software/hardware is necessary because of the breadth and speed at which the landscapes of the technology change. Therefore, this section will discuss the six categories of communication—Web 2.0, audio, video, creation tools, presentation tools, and learning object repositories—in general terms and provide commonly used programs. The most important rule when incorporating technology is to ensure that its use is appropriate to the learning objective and not being used just because it is "cool" and new.

Two technologies that span all of the outlined categories are mobile applications (apps) and tablet computing. The New Media Consortium (NMC) Horizon Report: Higher Education Edition (2013) outlines technologies that have a high probability of adoption within 1 year, 2 to 3 years, and 4 to 5 years. In the 2013 report, mobile apps and tablet computing are slated for adoption in 1 year or less. Since the opening of the first app store in July 2008 (by Apple, others came online shortly after) to September 2012, more than 55 billion apps have been downloaded and have found their way into almost every human endeavor (NMC Horizon Report, 2013). The report also details how mobile apps are useful in learning as they empower people to learn and experience new concepts regardless of location and via many devices. The second emerging technology, tablet computing, is seen as a growing competitive market. Tablets are adaptable to different environments, thousands of software options, lower cost than traditional laptops, and provide overall flexibility (NMC Horizon Report: 2013 Higher Education Edition).

Communication is the most important aspect of any course, as will be discussed in Chapter 8: Interacting and Communicating Online. The communication between the instructor and the class, the instructor and individual students, and student-to-student are vital to the online learning environment. Therefore, establishing communication avenues that are relevant to the course learning objectives, compatible with the technology infrastructure in place, and usable by the students is important. The three examples following are popular in the academic and corporate settings.

Web conferencing: Web conferencing surfaced in the late 1990s and is defined by PCMag.com (2013) as "a videoconferencing session via the Internet ... to interact with other participants, attendees use either a web application or an application downloaded into their client machines" (PCMag, 2013). As in a live classroom, web conferencing allows faculty and students to meet and collaborate with easy, real-time conversation exchanges with immediate feedback, as well as greater opportunities for faculty to alter the pace of the instruction and provide more opportunities for student assessment (Schullo, Hilbelink, Venable, & Barron, 2007). Many web conferencing systems allow for shared web browsing, file transfer, common whiteboard space, and chat. Common conferencing solutions are Blackboard Collaborate (previously Wimba and Elluminate), Cisco's Webex, Citrix's GoToMeeting, and Adobe Connect.

Instant Messaging: Instant messaging (IM) is defined by PCMag.com (2013) as the exchange of text messages in real-time (synchronous) between two or more people logged into a particular IM service. While IM has been around since the early 1990s and may seem like an outdated technology, it has evolved to still have a place in online learning by employing the use of many input devices, and by adding additional features that expand upon the PCMag definition. Most IM platforms allow users to communicate via their computer, cell phone, or other mobile device and some have expanded to allow features such as file sharing, audio messaging, and the use of avatars. IM can also be expanded into the use of a chat room, which allows multiple users to synchronously communicate in a common online area. Common IM solutions are AOL's Instant Messenger (AIM), ICQ, Yahoo! Messenger, Google Talk, Jabber, and Microsoft's MSN Messenger.

Discussion Boards: Discussion boards are also known as message boards, discussion groups, threaded discussions, bulletin boards, and online forums. They allow for an asynchronous conversation between two or more users through the use of posted text or audio messages. The messages usually follow an outline or tree composition with the overall structure being a forum, a topical conversation thread, or a single message post. When users respond to another user's post, the response is usually indented under the post to identify its relationship to other posts in the thread. A benefit of discussion boards over IM solutions is that the users do not need to be active in the environment at the same time, as messages are archived on the board for users to access when they are able. This benefit allows users to access messages on their schedule and provides them time to research and reflect in order to produce well-composed responses. While most LMSs have a discussion board capability built into the platform, some common stand-alone discussion board solutions are Google Groups, phpBB, and vBulletin.

The term Web 2.0 was introduced in 2004 and refers to technological improvements over what was previously available to allow a different level of user interaction. The three most common Web 2.0 technologies are blogs, wikis, and social networking. Betrus (2012) reported that more than 70% of introductory technology courses for pre-service teachers include the use of Web 2.0 technologies. Teachers report using Web 2.0 technologies to improve student learning, student-to-student interaction, student-to-instructor interaction, collaborative learning, and the sharing of content knowledge (Sadaf, Newby, & Ertmer, 2012).

The use of audio and video media is fast becoming as preferred by students as text-based materials. A distinct segment of students prefer audio material (such as podcasts) and videos to either digital or paper-based traditional learning materials (Robinson & Stubberud, 2012). One of the fastest growing fields is the use of webcasting. Sonic Foundry is an example of a webcasting platform that allows for the capture, management, and delivery of webcasts for online training, conference presentations, executive briefings, and academic course sessions. Sonic Foundry's Mediasite webcastings solution is currently used by more than 1,100 colleges and universities to broadcast or capture lectures (Sonic Foundry, 2013).

Faculty and students have the options to use many different types of tools for the creation and presentation of content. When deciding the best method to present or create material, it is important to remember that the technology used should be appropriate and related to the learning objective and not chosen because it's the newest technology. Some common, tried and true, creation and presentation technologies are:

- Google Docs: Google Docs allows users to create their work (documents, spreadsheets, surveys, etc.) online, work collectively, and easily share content with others (docs.google.com).
- YouTube: Allows users to upload original videos and to watch other users' videos on a wide array of topics (www.youtube.com/).

▪ Prezi and SlideRocket: Web applications that have the benefit of storing the presentation online, easily incorporating graphical elements and enhanced visual effects to aid in audience engagement (www.sliderocket.com and http://prezi.com).

▪ Tiki-Toki: A web application used to create interactive timelines (www.tiki-toki.com/).

▪ Visual.ly: A website with infographics and data visualizations. A user can either use the stored infographics on a variety of topics or create their own (visual.ly/).

Learning object repositories (LORs) are databases that house learning objects (LOs) and provide easy access to individual resources such as simulations, multimedia, animations, videos, or a combination of several materials to form modules, lessons, and many other types of objects that are discipline specific. LOs are educational content that use widely accepted specifications and standards that allows them to be searchable, interoperable, and reusable in different learning environments (McGreal, 2004). Frequently used LORs in academia are:

▪ Kahn Academy (www.khanacademy.org)
▪ MERLOT (www.merlot.org)
▪ NOVA (science resources; www.pbs.org/wgbh/nova/)
▪ TeacherTube (teachertube.com)
▪ University LORs (e.g., MIT Open Courseware, Texas A&M Digital Repository)
▪ State LORs (e.g., The Orange Grove, Florida's repository project)

A nursing specific LOR is Quality and Safety Education for Nurses (QSEN). QSEN's goal is to "preparing future nurses so that they will have the knowledge, skills, and attitudes (KSAs) necessary to continuously improve the quality and safety of the health care systems within which they work" and is a central repository for information on competencies, teaching strategies, and faculty development (QSEN, 2013).

STUDENT REQUIREMENTS

A student must have certain skills and have access to specific items in order to be a successful online learner. Nursing students have been found to lack knowledge of basic computer software, email and communication skills, and college-specific software related to traditional, hybrid, and online courses (Edwards & O'Connor, 2011). Some of the requirements to be an online student are basic, such as access to a computer and the Internet. These basic needs are communicated by the institution to the student as technical requirements. The technical requirements are specific to the needs of the school, the LMS, and other technologies the student will be required to use during the pursuit of a degree. An example of the technical requirements for the University of Maryland, School of Nursing can be found at nursing.umaryland.edu/nacs/resources-stud-pc-min. Other skills like a student's readiness to be an online learner and ability to use the LMS are not as easily measured, but equally important. There are basic and advanced online assessment tools that help students determine if online learning is a good fit for them and if they have the skills to be successful. A basic free quiz to determine if distance learning is appropriate for a student is offered by Red Deer College and can be found at www.rdc.ab.ca/future_students/high_school_students/distance_learning/Pages/SelfAssessmentQuiz.aspx. Smartmeasure.com is a more robust online assessment tool that is a "124-item assessment which measures a learner's readiness for succeeding in an online and/or technology rich learning program" and "indicates the degree to which an individual student possesses attributes, skills and knowledge that contribute to success in learning" (SmartMeasure, 2013). The site measures components in seven areas:

- Individual attributes: Motivation, procrastination, willingness to ask for help, and so forth
- Life factors
- Learning styles
- Technical competency
- Technical knowledge
- On-screen reading rate and recall
- Typing speed and accuracy

Students should also know how they learn best or their learning style. This information will help them determine if distance learning is a good fit for them and what resources they should seek. There are free online learning style inventories, such as the one offered at Edutopia.org (www.edutopia.org/multiple-intelligences-learning-styles-quiz Technical knowledge).

INSTRUCTOR REQUIREMENTS

An online instructor needs to have a different set of competencies than an instructor that only teaches in the traditional classroom. The most important of these competencies is to know that instructors must seek assistance in developing, designing, and planning for the technology used in their course. While many faculty are experts in the content and are talented teachers, "faculty members cannot be expected to know intuitively how to design and deliver an effective online course … seasoned faculty members have not been exposed to techniques and methods needed to make online work successful" (Palloff & Pratt, 2001, p. 23). The instructor must be able to adapt both the teaching style and the content in order to create the most advantageous learning environment for students. Nguyen, Zierler, and Nguyen (2011) surveyed 193 faculty members from nursing schools in the western United States and found that while 66% of faculty reported they were competent with distance-learning tools, 69% reported a need for additional training. Some of the required information is the same regardless of whether the instruction happens online or in a traditional classroom. Both modalities require the instructor to know the most up-to-date content, to know who the learners are, and how the course relates to the overall program. But the online instructor needs to have additional information and must overcome barriers specific to the online environment. Institutions, colleges, programs, and courses will have specific technology requirements of the instructor; therefore, it is important to think about necessary competencies in generalizable terms and not specific skills (e.g., expert in the use of Microsoft Office version 2010). Varvel (2007) composed a list of instructor competencies that is relevant and applicable to all online instructors (see Table 4.3).

In summary, LMSs continue to be hub on which institutions base their online learning, but a variety of accompaniments are being added to enhance the student experience and expand the instructor's toolbox for education. These accompaniments provide improved communication, increased collaboration, and the creation and distribution

TABLE 4.3   Technology Knowledge and Abilities

The competent instructor is knowledgeable about the technologies used in the virtual classroom (online classroom) and can make effective use of those technologies.

• Access: The competent instructor ...

  ° has access to the required technical equipment and software for the given medium and the course

  ° owns or has easy access to necessary technical equipment and software including a computer, a reliable Internet connection, and other equipment such as video editing that might be required by the given course and content

• Technical Proficiencies: The competent instructor ...

  ° is knowledgeable and has the ability to use computer programs that are typically required in online education to improve learning/teaching, personal productivity, and information management

  ° has an understanding of various commonly used web browsing softwares

  ° is proficient in the chosen course management system

  ° can modify content within the system as necessary

  ° can manage all student activities within the learning management system (LMS)

  ° has clear abilities within the primary communication channels of the LMS

  ° has the ability to use word processing software including the ability to compose documents using accessibility software as required

  ° has the ability to use and manage asynchronous and synchronous communication programs

  ° has a proficiency managing a computer operating system to maintain security updates, virus scanning software, and other software updates as necessary for the course

Source: Adapted from V. E. Varvel Jr. (2007). Master Online Teacher Competencies.

of high-quality audio/video learning objects. With the ever-expanding market for online education and technology, it is important to reinforce the true reason behind using any technology—to support the learner, instructor, and learning objectives at all levels. In order for the technology used to reach its maximum potential, instructors and students need to embrace the necessary competencies, be creative, and always be open to a new learning opportunity.

REFERENCES

Betrus, A. (2012). Historical evolution of instructional technology in teacher education programs: A ten-year update. *Techtrends: Linking Research & Practice to Improve Learning, 56*(5), 42–45. doi:10.1007/s11528-012-0597-x

Blackboard. (2013). About blackboard. Retrieved from http://www.blackboard.com/About-Bb

Catherall, P. (2008). Learning systems in post-statutory education. *Policy Futures in Education, 6*(1), 97–108.

Dunn, J. (2012). The 20 best learning management systems. Retrieved from http://edudemic.com/2012/10/the-20-best-learning-management-systems/

Edmodo. (2013). Features. Retrieved from http://www.edmodo.com/about

EduTools. (2013). CMS: Feature list. Retrieved February 01, 2013, from http://edutools.com/feature_list.jsp?pj=4

EduTools. (2013). EduTools homepage. Retrieved February 01, 2013, from http://edutools.com/index.jsp?pj=1

Edwards, J., & O'Connor, P. A. (2011). Improving technological competency in nursing students: The passport project. *Journal of Educators Online, 8*(2).

FindTheBest. (2013). Compare learning management systems. Retrieved from http://lms.findthebest.com/

Joomla. (2013). Learning management system comparison. Retrieved from http://www.joomlalms.com/compare/

McGreal, R. (Ed.). (2004). *Online education using learning objects.* Open and Distance Learning Series. London: Routledge/Falmer.

Moodle. (2013) About moodle. Retrieved from http://docs.moodle.org/24/en/About_Moodle

New Media Consortium, & EDUCAUSE Learning Initiative. (2013). NMC Horizon Report: 2013 Higher Education Edition. Retrieved from http://horizon.wiki.nmc.org/home

Nguyen, D. N., Zierler, B., & Nguyen, H. Q. (2011). A Survey of nursing faculty needs for training in use of new technologies for education and practice. *Journal of Nursing Education, 50*(4), 181–189. doi:http://dx.doi.org.proxy-hs.researchport.umd.edu/10.3928/01484834-20101130-06

Palloff, R., & Pratt, K. (2001). *Lessons from the cyberspace classroom: The realities of online teaching.* San Francisco, CA: Jossey-Bass.

PCMag.com. (2013). Retrieved from http:// www.pcmag.com

Piotrowski, M. (2009). Document-oriented e-learning components. *ERIC, EBSCOhost.* Retrieved January 30, 2013.

Quality and Safety Education for Nurses. (2013). About QSEN. Retrieved from http://qsen.org/about-qsen/

Robinson, S., & Stubberud, H. (2012). Student preferences for educational materials: Old meets new. *Academy of Educational Leadership Journal, 16,* 99–109.

Sadaf, A., Newby, T. J., & Ertmer, P. A. (2012). Exploring factors that predict preservice teachers' intentions to use web 2.0 technologies using decomposed theory of planned behavior. *Journal of Research on Technology in Education, 45*(2), 171–196.

Schullo, S., Hilbelink, A., Venable, M., & Barron, A. E. (2007). Selecting a virtual classroom system: Elluminate Live vs. Macromedia Breeze (Adobe Acrobat Connect Professional). *JOLT, 3.* Retrieved from http://jolt.merlot .org/vol3no4/hilbelink.htm

SonicFoundry. (2013). Why Mediasite by Sonic Foundry. Retrieved from http:// www.sonicfoundry.com/

Varvel Jr., V. E. (2007). Master online teacher competencies. *Online Journal of Distance Learning Administration, X*(I).

FIVE

Reconceptualizing the Online Course

CAROL A. O'NEIL

The stage between making the decision to use online learning strategies and actually developing the learning environment is most important. Reconceptualizing the learning material means going from, "Okay, I have this learning material," to using online pedagogy, infrastructure, and technology to make decisions about how the learning material will be presented online. Reconceptualizing is a series of "if-then" statements. It is a decision tree in which strengths, purposes, and resources are examined in order to make decisions concerning the best approach to use in presenting the learning material. Reconceptualizing is answering questions and using the answers to guide the development of online learning environments. The decision tree in Figure 5.1 will guide your decision making. It comprises questions, possible answers, and possible actions. Questions are posed about institutional issues, technology, faculty, and students. Possible answers to the questions are given, and actions based on each of the possible responses are proposed.

Institutional Issues

Questions	If	Then
What is the purpose of the learning material?	To support learning	Develop a hybrid or blended learning package
	To teach	Develop a full Web-based learning environment
How many students/nurses/consumers will engage in the learning?	More than 25	Divide into groups of 25 learners OR Consider hybrid/blended learning environment
	Less than 25	Consider offering fully online
How often will the learning be offered?	Short term (once or twice)/blended or hybrid	Form a team comprising content expert (CE), instructional designer (ID), and instructional technologist (IT), and consider which objectives can be best met online
	Long term (offered on regular basis)	Form a consortium of partners including CE, ID, IT and other support personnel and stakeholders to plan, prioritize, and develop
What is the financial impact?	Included in current budget	Follow established policies
	Needs financial support	Consider grant funding
		Gain outside support from private sources
		Consider a technology fee
What resources exist that you can access?	Within institution/local environment and minimal	Consider hybrid/blended learning
	Within institution/local environment and adequate or more than adequate	Assess your technology skills. Consider technology that can be used to most efficiently present material
	Resources available outside institution/local environment	Establish contracts, contacts, terms of use
What resources exist that you can join?	Institutional/local environment	Seek out resources, volunteer
	Campus/unit environment	Volunteer for committee
	System/community	Form collaborative partnership
What is the level of administrative support?	High	Review existing policies and gain needed approvals, i.e., curriculum committee
	Low	See immediate supervisor and discuss/estimate sources and amount of support
Is developing online material valued by administrators? Is it part of your job description/tenure, merit, and promotion?	Yes	Organize portfolio, document activities, and organize for peer review of course before and during initial pilot
	No	See immediate supervisor; teach course you are developing
Technology		
What institutional hardware and software are available to you?	Adequate bandwith and server	Strategic planing for developing and implementing courses
	Inadequate bandwidth and server	Consider partnerships; develop one online course
	Minimal software, no courseware	Contact vendors
	Adequate hardware and software	Engage in strategic planning actvities

(Continued)

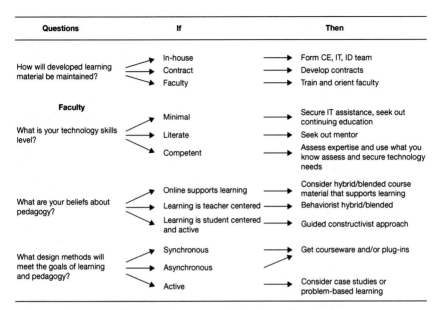

Questions	If	Then
How will developed learning material be maintained?	In-house Contract Faculty	Form CE, IT, ID team Develop contracts Train and orient faculty
Faculty What is your technology skills level?	Minimal Literate Competent	Secure IT assistance, seek out continuing education Seek out mentor Assess expertise and use what you know assess and secure technology needs
What are your beliefs about pedagogy?	Online supports learning Learning is teacher centered Learning is student centered and active	Consider hybrid/blended course material that supports learning Behaviorist hybrid/blended Guided constructivist approach
What design methods will meet the goals of learning and pedagogy?	Synchronous Asynchronous Active	Get courseware and/or plug-ins Consider case studies or problem-based learning

FIGURE 5.1 Reconceptualizing the online course.

USING THE DECISION TREE

The following is an example of how answering the decision tree questions can guide your decision making. A school of nursing is considering online courses. The dean meets with the department chair and a faculty member, Dr. G., who has experience in teaching online, to discuss the feasibility of moving the RN to BSN program online. The school has a strategic plan, developed with input from faculty, that includes online learning. This information about institutional factors leads to the conclusion that support for online programs is strong. The dean is willing to provide an information technology (IT) expert and instructional design (ID) support. The program will enroll more than 25 students and will be long term. The current budget will support development activities. No policies about online courses are available.

The school has its own server and enough bandwidth for courses. One instructional designer is available for consultation, but no maintenance support personnel are available. The school has 3-year-old desktop computers for faculty members. Microsoft Office® web development software is available. Several laptops are available to faculty and all computers have Internet access. Computer laboratories are available for students, with over 50 terminals in the school of nursing.

Dr. G. has been involved in a project to guide and mentor faculty to teach online for a year. She is computer literate and is a content expert (CE) in community health nursing. She believes that students learn through interacting with learning material and that students can learn from each other. Dr. G. believes that faculty motivates and guides learning. She would like to provide a variety of learning options for students. Dr. G. would like to include course content, discussions boards, small groups for students to complete activities, and synchronous meetings for office hours. She would like student assessment to include participation in discussions, assignments, and exam grades. Students should have computers available for use outside the school of nursing.

DECISIONS

Based on this information, one course in the RN to BSN program would be developed. This course would have a community focus, and Dr. G. would develop and teach it. Teaching the course would be included in her workload, and developing the course would be considered "service" and included as a "merit" activity. The current instructional designer would contract with a courseware vendor and would teach Dr. G. how to use the courseware. Dr. G. would partner with a technical person (IT) and the two would work as a CE and IT team. The course would be organized by modules; each module would have objectives, readings, content, small group activities, and large group discussion questions. Content would be disseminated in written and audio formats. Grading would include projects, participation, and exams.

The course is marketed prior to and at course registration and students register in the usual way. The names of the registered students were sent to Dr. G., and she entered the students into her online course. While the pilot was in process, the faculty administrator for the undergraduate program, Dr. G., and the instructional designer met to plan for future courses. Evaluation information from the pilot course was solicited several times during the course and at the end of the course, and was used to refine the course and to design other courses. One new course per faculty member was added each semester for a year. The lessons learned were shared with faculty who were developing their courses. The team guided and supported faculty developing and teaching new courses online. Faculty new to teaching online were invited to join the web-based teaching committee, and the team grew each semester. Sharing ideas and experiences with peers was essential for the development of the program. Through this group, policies, online student registration and support, and student and faculty support systems were developed.

Another possible scenario that might exist is high technical support and minimal faculty skill. If the faculty is motivated and willing to learn to develop online courses, go online. If there is moderate support and high resources, go online. If there is minimal support and resources, consider hybrid or blended courses and build support and stakeholders. A hybrid or blended course combines technology and traditional classroom strategies. Developing a hybrid or blended course is an excellent way to begin while gathering resources, support, and experience. Gravitate toward a level at which the effort will be successful. Maximize the resources available and incorporate new resources and technology that will enhance the course. Pilot the material, have the material peer reviewed, and solicit learner feedback frequently for incorporation into course revisions.

RECONCEPTUALIZING COURSES

Hybrid or Blended Courses

The administration decides to put a portion of the course material online. This is called "blended learning," which is defined as augmenting traditional face-to-face learning with technology. It is the mixing of technology with activities and interaction to create a seamless transition between learning and working. See Chapter 7 on blended learning.

What are some options for blended learning? Look at the learning goals and objectives, the available technology, and the skill level of the faculty. Think about maximizing the use of technology to create the most effective environment for student learning. Some of the options are:

- Use voice, video, text, or any combination thereof to put the essential content online. Class time could then be used for discussion activities and case studies. For example, narrate some didactic nursing class lectures to create a mini lecture using Microsoft PowerPoint® and RealPlayer®. Limit content to a specific unit of study; for example, depression. Give essential knowledge on depression that will accomplish the objectives, limiting the learning material to about 20 minutes. The required reading on depression and the mini lecture on depression should be completed before class. Use in-class time for small group discussion of case studies. The case studies will help the student to begin to apply the content. Use the scenario of depression in a teenager, a postpartum woman, or an adult. Care plans can be the outcome of the case studies.

- Use class time to impart content and use online environments to support learning through links relevant to the learning material.
- Use online support for administrative and organizational functions such as grading, computerized examinations, announcements, directions, and syllabus presentation. Use the online environment for discussion of case studies. Set up a discussion forum for each case study or divide the students into small groups to discuss the case study and develop care plans.

Mental Models

Once the decision to present the learning material online is made, the next step is to develop plans that will maximize the available resources, including hardware and software. It is more effective to use what is available to its optimal capacity and to use what is known to the fullest potential to produce a learning environment that will maximize assets. The "lowest common denominator" should be attained, which means that not all students have access to the same hardware and software. If a course is built using software that the student does not have or does not have access to, the student will become frustrated and dissatisfied. For example, when using a mini lecture requiring plug-ins for viewing multimedia or audio files, the content of this mini lecture may not be available to students with older computers or slow dialup connections. Providing content using links and text will provide information to a larger audience because it is the lowest common denominator and the most accessible to students.

How can the course instructor convert traditional learning material to an online learning environment? What may be used to create the online learning environment? These are the next questions in reconceptualizing online learning environments. Because of the lack of visual feedback from students (shaking of heads while you are lecturing or closed eyes and bobbing heads), the online learning environment needs to give students a clear picture of what they are learning and how they will learn it. In the traditional classroom, the teacher begins a learning session by telling the students what they will learn (learning objectives), gives them the information needed to learn the content, and then summarizes what the students have learned. A traditional teacher begins by saying "Today we are going to learn about depression" and at the end of the discussion might say, "Let me summarize what we have said about depression," so the students know where they are in the learning process. In online learning environments, students still need to know where they are in the learning process but this is done through mental models. Mental models give meaning to concepts and promote the transfer of knowledge from the "didactic" to the "real" world.

EXAMPLE OF RECONCEPTUALIZING ONLINE LEARNING ENVIRONMENTS

Let us follow Dr. G. in the reconceptualization process. Dr. G. reconceptualized an undergraduate Community/Public Health Nursing course. She considered her pedagogical beliefs that students learn differently and have unique learning styles. She decided to include learning strategies such as text, verbal, and discussion modes of learning to accommodate a variety of learning styles. Dr. G. decided to organize the content by modules. The traditional classroom course was organized by "week"—Week 1, Week 2, and so forth. The online course includes objectives and readings, content, and small group activities. The content outline looks like this:

Community/Public Health Nursing

Module 1: History of Community/Public Health Nursing
- Objectives and Readings
- Content
- Activities

Module 2: Influences on the Practice of Community/Public Health Nursing
- Objectives and Readings
- Content
- Activities

Module 3: Cultural Influences on the Practice of Community/Public Health Nursing
- Objectives and Readings
- Content
- Activities

This organizing framework continued to Module 15 for a 15-week course. This design was cumbersome and needed streamlining. Dr. G. looked at the content and decided that the course really contained four areas of content: History and Scope, Practice, Focus, and Tools. Dr. G. shifted the modules into four content areas as illustrated in Figure 5.2.

Each section contains several of the original modules. History and Scope comprises Modules 1, 2, and 3; Practice comprises Modules 4, 5, 6, and 7; Focus comprises Modules 8 and 9; and Tools comprises Modules 10, 11, and 12. The content areas and the modules within that area are presented in the same color and each content area has a different color. Each module contains objectives and readings, mini-lectures, podcasts, and activities. This reconceptualization has several advantages. Students repeatedly see the four content areas, and these become the four concepts of Community/Public Health Nursing. The concepts, called "mental models," are consistently reinforced when the student accesses the course content. Mental models give meaning to concepts and promote the transfer of knowledge from the "didactic" to the "real" world. When the student sees the word "Tools" over and over, the student forms a mental model that community/public health nursing has tools, and one of those tools is epidemiology (a module). Operationalizing the mental model in an activity strengthens the impact of the mental model. For example,

History and Scope	Focus
Practice	Tools

FIGURE 5.2 The reconceptualized course.

one of the activities in the Tools mental model could include a case study of an epidemic of influenza in a community. Reconceptualizing a course provides students with a "map" of the course so they can see what the course is about, where they have been, and where they are going in the course.

Pedagogy

First consider the pedagogical beliefs and think about what can be used to operationalize those beliefs. Ask yourself the following questions:

- Do you prefer one learning style or many?
- Do you believe that group communication will support learning?
- Do you support synchronous communication?
- Do you support asynchronous communication?

The technology to be used to create the course is the next decision. Some options are audio, video, links, podcasts, wikis, text, or PowerPoint presentations. Start with what is familiar and consider the preferred philosophy of teaching and learning.

Example of Reconceptualizing Pedagogy

Consider how Dr. G. operationalizes her philosophical and pedagogical beliefs about teaching and learning online. Dr. G. chose to include mini-lectures with voice-synchronized PowerPoint. The mini lecture included content that was pertinent to meeting the module objectives and to complete the module activities. The voice scripts were included in print, and both the PowerPoint slides and the scripts were available to students, thus allowing for a wider variety of learning styles using voice and text. Students are divided into small groups to complete module activities. Students post ideas to a discussion board, which contains a question relating each module to the real world. An example of a small group activity is as follows: Students are given census data about a geographic community. They also view a video tour of the same community. Students are asked to develop a consensus "composite picture" of the community using both types of data. Each group can post its composite picture on the discussion board. Dr. G. provides synchronous office hours for 1 hour a week.

Another consideration is grading. Will participation be graded? If so, how does the student need to participate to earn a grade? Traditionally, schools of nursing are bound by approval of the curriculum committee. Do traditional and online classes have the same syllabus? Must grading be the same with both modalities? If so, how will participation be included in the online learning environment? Is grading of participation necessary to engage students in active communication during the course? Participation can be a mandatory and expected behavior in online courses. (Examples of criteria for expected participation and grading can be found in Chapter 9: Course Management Methods.)

Reconceptualizing Laboratory Courses

Because many nursing courses have associated laboratory experiences, consideration must be made for learning psychomotor skills. The components of the learning process for psychomotor skills that differ in traditional versus online learning environments are practice and feedback. Traditional learners learn the procedure then attend laboratory sessions to perform the skill under the supervision of an expert, who in turn will give the students feedback on their performance. Once they master the skill in the laboratory, the student will perform the skill with a proctor and their proficiency will be evaluated. Another name for this clinical activity is called a "cognitive apprenticeship," which is discussed in further detail in Chapter 8 on interaction. Students learning in online environments can obtain the didactic material online. The challenge is to provide students with practice opportunities, feedback, and evaluation. Some options are:

- Online students attend the laboratory sessions with traditional students.
- Instructors assign preceptors in the community for the students, and the preceptor gives feedback to the student.
- Students choose preceptors, and the instructor coordinates and monitors the experience while the preceptor gives feedback.
- Clinical instructors can be assigned to a geographic cohort of students; the laboratory experience is contracted with local institutions and the instructor gives feedback to the students.
- Partner with schools of nursing and contract for use of their laboratory facilities and obtain feedback from instructors.

- Use laptops or iPads with videoconferencing ability to practice skills with the instructor at a remote location, who then gives feedback.

Some options for assessing students are:

- Students can take a proficiency test administrated by the instructor at the school of nursing.
- The proficiency test can be given and assessed by the preceptor.
- The proficiency test can be administered by a preceptor, video-taped, and then assessed by the instructor.
- The student can take the proficiency test at an outreach site where an instructor will administer and assess students in a geographic cohort.
- Community resources can administer the proficiency test at an outreach site, and the instructor can assess student proficiency via live video.
- Students can use a laptop computer and videoconferencing to perform the proficiency test, with the instructor assessing from a remote site.

Reconceptualizing Clinical Courses

Some courses that are offered online have a clinical component. Clinical experiences should provide the students with guidance, mentoring, role modeling, feedback, and assessment of clinical competencies associated with the course. The following questions should be asked:

- How will guidance and mentoring be given to the student and by whom?
- Who will provide role modeling and how?
- How will the student receive feedback?
- How will the mastery of course competencies be assessed for each student?

Some suggestions for providing clinical students with guidance, mentoring, and role modeling are:

- Distance learning students enroll in the same clinical experiences as traditional students. If students are location bound, other clinical options must be developed.

- Students have a faculty-appointed or student-selected preceptor who acts as a role model and who provides students with experiences to accomplish the clinical objectives.
- Students have clustered experiences—the instructor arranges for geographically clustered, intensive experiences, (e.g., 4-day, 32- to 40-hour experiences for a cohort of students in a specific geographic location).

Videoconferencing with the instructor provides student-to-student and student-to-instructor interactions. The student can answer questions, and the faculty can observe student performance or student patient interactions and give feedback. Logs written by students in location-bound settings and shared with the preceptor and instructor provide information for the instructor to assess student perception and progress toward meeting clinical objectives.

In summary, reconceptualizing the learning environment begins with the decision to transfer traditional course material into an online learning environment. The process of answering questions about a course and using the answers to guide the development of the online learning and communication environments will help capitalize on the benefits of the web and computer technology. Many opportunities exist to enhance an online course through the appropriate application of technology, such as multimedia, links, and synchronous and asynchronous discussions. Laboratory and clinical courses are challenges for designing nursing courses in an online format, but as the technology advances, current methods of offering these courses can only be improved.

SIX

Designing the Online Environment

CAROL A. O'NEIL

Instructional design refers to a systematic and reflective process that translates the principles of learning and instruction (the pedagogy) into plans for instructional materials, activities, information resources, and evaluation (Smith & Ragan, 2004). Instructional design answers the questions: Where are we going? How will we get there? How will we know when we get there? Smith and Ragan (2004) identified three components in the instructional design process:

- Instructional analysis (Where are we going?)
- Instructional strategy (How will we get there?)
- Evaluation (How will we know when we get there?)

Instructional *analysis* includes assessing the learner and developing learning goals and objectives. Instructional *strategy* includes developing, delivering, and maintaining the methods and strategies for learning. *Evaluation* includes using strategies to assess the student's progress toward attaining the objectives (Smith & Ragan, 2004). The design should be specific enough so that it is easy to implement, but flexible enough to allow faculty to be creative.

Instructional design theory provides guidance in developing learning environments. Instructional design is the preparation and production of learning material and includes developing objectives and goals and formulating teaching and assessment strategies. Educational theory guides design structure.

ELEMENTS OF DESIGN

The Center for Teaching and Faculty Development (San Francisco State University) suggested key principles for the universal design of learning. One of the main principles is that faculty represents course concepts and engagement in a variety of ways, which will allow students to express what they have learned. Several terms are used: *representation*, which is the design and delivery of learning; *engagement*, which is the students' active participation in the course; and *expression*, which is how the students demonstrate their learning.

The term "guided constructivism" is often used in learning design. It is a combination of elements from behaviorist and constructivist theories. Behaviorism is reflected in the use of objectives that are behaviorally stated, measurable, and timed. Constructivism employs active learning strategies to engage students in the learning process through interaction and meaningful learning.

The purpose of the constructivist learning environment is to provide learning opportunities in which students construct new knowledge based on existing knowledge and experience. The learning environment should be safe, supportive, and motivating so that learners can interact, solve real-world problems, work collaboratively and meaningfully, and assess their learning (Brandon, 2004). The role of the designer is to provide the appropriate learning environment so that learners can accomplish this purpose.

In this chapter, guided constructivist theory will be used to design learning environments for nursing. Constructivists view learning as student centered and advocate that learning objectives be developed by the learner. Although this is feasible for many disciplines, it is not always feasible for nursing. Nursing relies on learning objectives that are generated by the instructor. Objectives must be included in the design of nursing courses and will most likely be instructor generated—a characteristic of behaviorist theory. Combining instructor-driven objectives with the constructivist view results in what is called guided constructivism. Using the constructivist approach, the target population, interaction will be discussed. The design considerations will include:

- The target population
- The purpose and objectives
- Course organization
  - Content
  - Designs
  - Activities
  - Developing multimedia
- Navigation
- Page layout
- Interaction
  - Synchronous
  - Asynchronous
  - Discussion questions

THE TARGET POPULATION

The first step in course design is assessing the learners (the target population), their existing knowledge of the course material, their experience in learning in online environments, and their level of computer competence. For example, an undergraduate nursing course introducing new students to the concepts of health would be structured differently from a senior level course in community health nursing with a clinical component. The new students may be RNs returning to school for the first time in many years. This may be the first online course some learners have taken, so they have no experience with learning online. Their technical skills may be weak, and they probably do not know other students in the course or program. On the other hand, the senior level students may already have had a required technology course. They may have either taken or heard about online courses from other students, so they have a support group. They may be assigned to a clinical group with a clinical instructor who can answer questions and clarify the content that is learned online. The design for the new student would be more structured with explicit due dates for activities than for the senior student.

To increase socialization among new students, small groups might be organized so students can share their ideas with five or six other students instead of the larger class. Because participation is so important to the learning process, including a grade for participation in the class is a consideration. The discussion questions would be structured differently in each class. The new students may or may not be nurses, so discussion questions might incorporate life experiences to which all students can relate. The new students may be asked to devise a composite picture of a healthy community based on their readings and personal experiences, whereas the seniors might be asked to develop a nursing care plan for a multiproblem family or for pregnant teens in a community. The RN to BSN students tend to use nursing lingo that the traditional BSN (non-RN) student may not understand. In a discussion about using the Health Belief Model to develop a colon cancer prevention program, the RNs may be discussing colonoscopies while the non-RNs are asking, "What's that?" If the new student class comprises all RN to BSN students, the activities can be devised to incorporate nursing experience. Ask yourself who are the learners, what are their experiences with online learning, and what do they know about the learning material.

Assessing learning style is also important for the designer and the learner. The instructor or course designer can provide a variety of learning activities that address the different modes of learning. The VARK, Learning Style Inventory, Multiple Intelligences, and the Myers-Briggs Type Indicator outlined in Chapter 2, "Pedagogy Associated With Learning in Online Environments," are assessment resources.

Consideration should be given to how the learner moves through the learning experience. Learning can be self-paced, where the learner independently progresses through the learning experience. Alternatively, learners can be admitted to a series of courses or learning experiences at the same time (as a cohort). The cohort takes courses on the same schedule and ends the courses at the same time. Consider which will be more effective for your learners.

THE PURPOSE

The purpose of the learning experience should be stated in general terms and should resemble goals. From the goals should flow the objectives. Objectives should be stated in measurable terms and should succinctly communicate what the student will accomplish by the end of the learning experience. Objectives should be learner and content appropriate. Objectives for the course may be broadly outlined in the course syllabus, but should be broken down into manageable objectives for the learning content. For example, a course objective may be that the learner will plan, implement, and evaluate a smoking cessation program in a community group. In the learning module, this broad objective is broken down into smaller objectives, for example "The learner will describe the process of developing an implementation plan" or "The learner will define formative evaluation."

COURSE ORGANIZATION

The course organization is dependent on the content and the learners, and answers the question: What is the best way to present the content for the learners to learn? There is no right or wrong method, but what is important is having a rationale for making decisions. The design should be easy to navigate, logical, and structured, so that content builds on content previously delivered in the course.

CONTENT

Content is the information the learner needs to know to successfully achieve the objectives. Considering that learners have many different learning styles, the content should be presented using many different strategies. You may question, "Why?" The answer is, "Because we can!"—we can easily present content using different formats. Some examples of instructional formats to present content are: audio files, newspaper or journal articles, movie clips, videos, guest speakers, interactive software, links, interviews, or text-based materials.

There are two steps to organizing content. First, break the content into "chunks" (also called scaffolding) and then organize the chunks. The chunks can be logical units or delivered in a hierarchy of importance. A hierarchy can be used to structure relationships among chunks. Chunks should be logical and organized, for example, in modules or units. These chunks of information are then organized into a flexible and logical format, and then are organized into mental models. Mental models show the learner what they are learning, where they are in the course, and the relationship of each chunk in the course to other chunks of information. For example, an undergraduate course in gerontological nursing may be divided into the following chunks or modules:

Module 1: Introduction to the aging process
Module 2: Theories of aging
Module 3: Physical, psychological, sociological, and spiritual aspects of aging
Module 4: Common health problems
Module 5: Assessing the client
Module 6: Assessing the family
Module 7: Interventions: Needs and resources
Module 8: Legal issues related to aging
Module 9: Ethical issues related to aging

These chunks should be then organized into mental models. One approach is to combine Modules 1 to 3 into a section that called "The aging process." Modules 4 to 7 could be called "Caring for the aging client and family." The final section could be "Considerations in nursing care" (Modules 8 and 9). The mental models could be the aging process, caring for aging clients, and considerations in nursing care. When the learner navigates to Module 1, the learner must pass through "The aging process," thus illustrating where the learner is in the course and what is next in the course. The repetition of the mental models will instill in the student that in gerontological nursing, the nurse assesses and implements nursing care with the client and family, and, finally, the characteristics of the aging process and legal and ethical issues should be considered in nursing care.

DESIGN

Once the content is conceptualized, the next step is to decide how to structure the course. Course material is usually linked from the home page so it is easy to navigate. Discrete chunks of information are organized from the home page by using banners across the top and bottom and a menu bar down the left side. Every chunk should be relevant and meaningful to the learner. The most common left-side menu chunks are: course information, assignments, learning content, and discussion area. The design should provide a predetermined structure that will guide the learner through the learning environment. This design adds a structure that will help novice users navigate the materials, and seasoned users to know where to look for information. A disadvantage is that navigating is limited to forward and backward with the home page as the organizing point.

ACTIVITIES

Activities support learner progression through the content material. Activities should include real-world experiences and active learning strategies. Some activities are: case studies, group or individual projects, peer interaction through discussion, and active learning strategies such as collaborative problem solving.

MULTIMEDIA

Resources and experience help determine the use of multimedia presentations. Most instructors stay with what they know and what they have, because, in general, instructors do not have the time or technical skill to develop their own multimedia presentations. There is little or no information in the literature to give guidance whether a multimedia presentation is more effective than a text-based presentation of content. However, multimedia does offer an alternative way of learning for those students who prefer audio presentations.

The general rule of thumb is that "less is more." In other words, instructors can sometimes overuse technological enhancements, which end up not enhancing the course or content at all. If overused or used incorrectly, multimedia presentations can be distracting. Animation, for example, can be effectively used to demonstrate the flow of blood through the chambers of the heart, but it can also be used inappropriately, causing your course to resemble a Las Vegas billboard.

NAVIGATION

Using the three-click rule will help with organizing the flow of information. Get the learner where you want them to go in three clicks of the mouse. Navigation directions can be in the form of a graphic, a picture, or text. Regardless of which is used, be consistent and place the same thing in the same location on every page. Whether it is text along the left side of the page, or text boxes strung across the bottom of the page, or icons in the center of the page and text at the bottom, continue this pattern on every page. The home link is most important in navigation, because it gets the learner back to a central place. Some "do not's" are:

- Do not overuse bolding. It causes confusion.
- Do not use the color blue to emphasize text because blue is associated with hypertext.
- Do not use more than three different fonts, because this may confuse the learner.

Penn State Learning Design Community Hub (ets.tlt.psu.edu/learningdesign/) offers resources on learning objectives, multimedia, storyboarding, and navigating.

PAGE LAYOUT

Consistency means using the same layout on each page; this includes color, background, fonts, headings, text layout, and navigation cues. The graphic design should be fun, professional, simple, high tech, and slick. The design is a reflection of the organization and should be professional, of course, but also functional and easy to use. Too much information on a page can make the page look cluttered and can interfere with what the learner should learn. Ask yourself how each piece of information on a page will help the learner learn.

The basic page layout includes links that are color coded and positioned in the same place on every page. Each page should have a title at the top that describes what is on the page. Here are some additional tips on page layout:

▨ Use headings, bolding, bullets, and graphics to emphasize important information and use them consistently.

▨ Group information into logical units or chunks and be consistent in the groupings.

▨ Look at each page through the eyes of the learner and visualize the flow of information.

The home page should include information that the learner needs to begin the learning process. The vital data that should be on the home page are a link to course information, instructor information, communication, assignments, a welcome message from the instructor, and the required textbook and how to obtain it.

INTERACTING

Synchronous interaction requires participation with others at the same time, such as web conferencing. Asynchronous interactions such as bulletin boards, wikis, and blogs are not time dependent. Students should have several ways of asynchronous interactions. There should be a forum in which learners introduce themselves. This can be based on a general question such as "What would you like to tell us about yourself?," or something more specific, such as "When did you realize that you wanted to be a nurse?" for first-year nursing students. The introductory forum provides an opportunity for learners to find out what they have in common. If it is possible, learners should provide pictures of themselves and the instructor should provide a picture as well. These activities enhance bonding and start building learning communities. The second interaction is related to obtaining help for technology and course questions. Student questions should be answered by the instructor of the technical support team. The third type of interaction is a content forum, which is used to discuss experiences with the course material. The fourth is a student lounge, used for discussions not related to the course.

Discussion questions should be used to stimulate interaction among students and instructors. These questions should be open ended and based on the relevant course content. They should stimulate student thinking and facilitate students learning from each other.

For example, "How would you apply the principles from Unit 1 to your area of interest in nursing?" When done correctly, the answers to discussion questions will end in yet another question, thereby bringing the discussion to a higher level. For example, the student may end by saying, "Have others had a different experience?" Often it is necessary for the instructor to model this type of answer by offering his/her own experiences for the students to follow.

MODELS OF DESIGN

"A Course Design Model," developed by Margaret Chambers, Director of the Institute of Distance Education at the University of Maryland University College and the Web Initiative in Teaching Project instituted by the University System of Maryland from 1998 to 2002, outlines the following phases and components:

Phase One

Mapping: Identify goals, issues, and constraints

Architecture: Reconceptualize the course and restructure it into modules or educational objects

Prototype: Design a sample learning module illustrating the design decisions

Phase Two

Early development: Develop key elements, modules, or educational objects for testing with students

Field testing: Try out critical elements with real students and colleagues

Late development: Complete courseware

Phase Three

Institutional launch: Arrange for course listing, marketing, and registration; post a course review site

Pilot course delivery: Teach the course online with external peer reviewers

Revision: Modify and update

Storyboarding provides a method for designing an online course. It is a visual display that outlines the course and structure (Varvel, 2004). Quality Matters (QM) is a "faculty-centered, peer review process that is designed to certify the quality of online and blended courses" (Quality Matters, 2010). One component of the program is the QM Rubric, which consists of indicators of a quality online course. Although it is an evaluation program, the indicators can be used as a guide in developing a new course. For example, one indicator of a quality course is objectives and the indicator is that the objectives are measurable and fit the purpose of the course. For more information, consult the Quality Matters website and rubric.

SUMMARY

Design begins with an assessment of the learner and the technological expertise of the developer. Begin design with behavioral objectives that are appropriate to the learner and based on the content. The structure is dependent on the learning platform, but regardless of the "givens," multiple methods of learning should be included to accommodate various student learning styles. The learner can navigate via graphics or text, but should be able to get where he/she wants to go in three clicks (or less) of the mouse. The layout of every page should be identical and follow a template so the learner knows where he/she is on a page and how to navigate elsewhere. Learners need to communicate with each other and with the instructor. The most common form of communication is through discussion boards, but there are other means of interacting, such as through web conferences.

REFERENCES

Brandon, B. (2004, June 29). Applying instructional systems processes to constructivist learning environments. *The eLearning Developers' Journal.* Retrieved from http://www.elearningguild.com/pdf/2/062904DES.pdf

Quality Matters. (2010). Retrieved from http://www.qmprogram.org

San Francisco State University. The Center for Teaching and Faculty Development. Retrieved from http://ctfd.sfsu.edu/udl.htm

Smith, P. L., & Ragan, T. J. (2004). Instructional design. New York: John Wiley & Sons. The Center for Teaching and Faculty Development. Retrieved from http://ctfd.sfsu.edu/udl.htm

Varvel, V. E. (2004). Using storyboards in online course design. Retrieved from http://www.ion.uillinois.edu/resources/pointersclickers/2004_09/index.asp

SEVEN

Blended Learning

MATTHEW J. RIETSCHEL AND KATHLEEN M. BUCKLEY

The term "blended learning" is often used interchangeably with other terms in educational and research realms. Blended learning is also referred to as hybrid learning, mixed mode learning, web-enhanced instruction, technology-enhanced instruction, and technology-mediated instruction. In recent years, the term blended learning has been used with more regularity and is becoming the accepted term for education that combines face-to-face instruction with computer-mediated activities. Blended learning has been found to combine the best elements of traditional and online learning; it is likely to progress and become more dominant than either model alone (Watson, 2008). Allen, Seamen, and Garrett (2007) define blended courses and programs as having between 30% and 79% of content delivered online (technology-mediated) and the remainder delivered in a traditional, face-to-face environment. Technology-mediated instruction occurs with users in different physical locations, and the face-to-face instruction occurs in the same physical space. Staker and Horn (2012) define blended learning as "a formal education program in which a student learns at least in part through online delivery of content and instruction with some element of student control over time, place, path, and/or pace and at least in part at a supervised brick-and-mortar location away from home" (p. 3).

While the definition specifically speaks to the K–12 environment, it is quite applicable to higher education as well.

The blended learning approach can occur at the course level, the programmatic level, or the institutional level. At the course level, the blending of delivery modes occurs for a single subject over the span of one semester. At the programmatic level, the blended approach can occur within a course or across courses in a program; selected courses may be completely online while others are taught in a traditional face-to-face format. At an institutional level, the blended model can be expanded so that an institution uses a blended approach to deliver all of its course offerings. The last approach is used by most of the state virtual school supplemental online programs (e.g., Michigan Virtual School), by national district programs, and some consortium programs such as the Massachusetts-based Virtual High School Global Consortium (Watson & Gemin, 2010).

ORGANIZING THE DELIVERY AND CONTENT

Blended learning is not traditional face-to-face instruction and it is not online learning; it is its own instructional strategy and therefore needs to be approached differently than other formats. As articulated in Chapter 5 on reconceptualization, the delivery format and repertoire of learning tools need to be addressed when going through the process of reconceptualization and designing a course. This is especially true when approaching blended learning. Blended learning has the opportunity to take on endless forms, so the relationship between content and delivery needs to be carefully planned. It would be a disservice to students, faculty, and the institution for a traditionally classroom-based course or a fully online course to use the same educational approaches and content in a blended learning approach.

Delivery Formats

There are a variety of delivery formats becoming available for blended learning. The most common include face-to-face, in-class sessions on campus coupled with online activities. In many programs web conferencing is also becoming a part of the blended format, where students are able to meet via cameras and microphones to interact in real time from a distance.

Scheduling of Delivery Formats

Most blended programs have a pre-set schedule of delivery formats in order to coordinate students coming to campus for several courses during the same period of time. For example, students may be scheduled to attend in-class sessions the first and last weeks of the semester with online course work and periodic web conferencing sessions making up the balance of course delivery formats over the rest of the semester. Schedules are usually developed and circulated to the students prior to the start of the semester, so that they are able to plan their professional and personal responsibilities around class meetings on campus or via web conferencing. Fitting the content within a pre-set schedule of delivery format may require some adjustment in the organization of course content.

Maximizing the Delivery Format

In a classroom-based course, the content may usually be covered in a set order, such as one that may mimic the order of the chapters in the accompanying textbook. However, it is not always possible for the content to be covered in its natural order, as the schedule for the different modes of delivery may be set by the school or program. These schedules are often driven by days and times most convenient to the student population to be able to attend face-to-face or online synchronous sessions, distance-learning students who may have to travel to attend on-campus classes, availability of meeting spaces, and the need for technical or specialized support. For example, personnel may only be available on certain days and times to cover instructional activities in a clinical simulation environment, or online activities may need to be scheduled around known downtime for the online technology platform.

If the schedule is pre-set for a blended course, instructors should consider how to best match the content and approaches with delivery format. This can be done by mapping the delivery formats against module objectives, content to be covered, instructional strategies, and methods of assessment and evaluation. See Figure 7.1 for an example of mapping for a Nursing Informatics course consisting of online learning combined with in-class and web conferencing sessions. The faculty should place a high priority on maintaining curricular integrity and quality during this planning process to ensure that content delivered via web-based formats meet the same academic standard of

Course Delivery Format	Module Objectives	Content	Activities	Evaluation
In-class session	Module 1: Information Theories and Models • Discern the relevance of informatics to DNP practice • Analyze the Data, Information, Knowledge and Wisdom (D-I-K-W) model and other theories used in informatics practice • Evaluate the relevance of the D-I-K-W model in health care technology and student's specific area of interest	Nursing science and its relationship to nursing roles and nursing informatics Introduction to Data, Information, Knowledge and Wisdom (D-I-K-W) model Transforming nursing practice through technology	Required readings Class discussion	In-class participation and verbal feedback from peers and faculty
Online session	Module 2: The Model: Data, Information, Knowledge, Wisdom? • Evaluate how information technology impacts nursing practice • Assess how information technologies impact the role of nurses as knowledge workers • Develop recommendations to improve the system for use by nurses	Overview of Nursing Informatics How health information technologies impact nursing practice	Readings Discussion board question	Discussion Board Participation rubric

Course Delivery Format	Module Objectives	Content	Activities	Evaluation
Online session	Module 3: Information Science – The Foundation of Knowledge • Categorize the types of knowledge provided by a real-world information system or technology • Decide how that knowledge may generate practice wisdom • Describe how data from one information system create information that generates knowledge, which builds wisdom and influences nursing practice	How information systems generate knowledge that influences nursing practice	Required readings Student group work via web conferencing outside of class meetings with posting of group response on Course Discussion Board	Group Assignment rubric
Web conferencing session	Module 4: Selecting and Evaluating an Information System • Identify the *Systems Development Life Cycle* as the best practice process for system implementation • Support the value of the DNP role in the Life Cycle Process • Construct a potential plan for evaluation of the system	Selection and evaluation of an information system The *Systems Development Life Cycle* and the nursing role	Required readings Interview of user engaged in implementation of health care information system Sharing of interview results and discussion via web conferencing class	Participation in web conferencing group discussion and verbal feedback from peers and faculty

FIGURE 7.1 Mapping of course delivery format.

excellence as the face-to-face format. To follow the same order in the blended format may underutilize the available course delivery mode. Attention should be given to making sure that the delivery format is being used to its best advantage. The best case is when the content drives the delivery format, as this allows for the greatest use of available resources.

Classroom-Based Sessions

When deciding how best to use classroom-based sessions, faculty may consider these as excellent opportunities for community building. Palloff and Pratt (2007) regard social presence as a critical element in community building. Social presence theory, developed by Short, Williams, and Christie (1976), has been defined as the degree to which people are perceived as being real persons rather than objects. It is reinforced by communicating with other participants in a course not only through physical indicators such as eye contact, body language, and a projection of interest or excitement, but also through exchanges of information via dialogue. When possible, holding the first class as a face-to-face, classroom-based session allows an instructor to take maximum advantage of this type of communication among students to reinforce social presence and bonding (Ackerman, 2008a). However, spending the session lecturing on a particular topic or focusing on the mechanics of a course management system does little to reinforce establishing a relationship among faculty and students, and minimizes the opportunity for community building. Activities to encourage social presence should be carefully planned.

Introductions are an easy way to begin the first session, giving faculty and students the ability to closely view the physical person though their mannerisms, gestures, voice tone and quality, and all that goes into making them unique persons, while taking in the information that they are sharing about themselves. Introductions might be followed by learning activities that encourage students not only to interact, but also to create opportunities for sharing and collaborative learning. Being able to manipulate the physical environment easily is another advantage of on-campus, face-to-face meetings. Small-group work is relatively easy in this kind of setting. Students can be asked to quickly rearrange themselves in groups and discuss a series of questions on the content, work on a case study, or review and critique evidence-based articles. Engagement through these kinds of activities is the first step toward building a sense of comfort and security among students, which helps them to achieve self-confidence, a necessary component of collaboration (Ackerman, 2008b).

Many programs schedule the last class as a face-to-face, on-campus session. This time is often used for student presentations as a means to evaluate their understanding of the content. However, viewing multiple, back-to-back student presentations can quickly burn out the audience with little learning occurring. With the availability of web conferencing, presentations can now be recorded by students and posted for viewing asynchronously by the instructor and their peers. A final class session can then be used for more in-depth discussion of the presentations that have already been viewed. With the current ease in recording, there is no longer any need to use classroom time for watching presentations. It may be of greater value to schedule an in-class session earlier in the term and use it for activities that are best accomplished face-to-face.

Online Delivery

The online delivery format allows for a multitude of other learning activities, depending on the features of the available course management system. Community building can continue with other delivery modes. A blended course, when compared to a fully online or a traditional course, can lead to a stronger sense of learner community and higher learning scores (Rovai & Jordan, 2004). Faculty should carefully prepare to take advantage of any instructional technologies that are available that may encourage interaction among students and continue to build the community of learning. These interactive activities may include discussion board questions, wikis, blogs, or the posting of voice/video threads (Adelman & Nogueras, 2013). Because there is a greater risk of students experiencing feelings of isolation in the online environment, technology that supports social presence helps learners feel a more personal and emotional connection as part of a community.

Web Conferencing

Web conferencing offers another dimension of being able to interact "face-to-face" as in a classroom but via the Internet and the use of audio-video technology. With classroom-based discussion, there is the advantage of giving and receiving immediate feedback, which may create an illusion in which the technology almost disappears and participants have the sense of being together in the same place. The best use of this delivery format is again not with a lecture—lectures can be videotaped and placed in online modules for convenient and repeated viewing. The opportunity for interaction should be optimized with group activities and discussions. One superior advantage of this delivery format is being able to bring guest experts who are at a distance to the sessions. In a classroom-based course, because of the expense and inconvenience, it may be impossible for students to meet with these experts, but with web conferencing the only things needed are the expert's willingness, time for the session itself, and access to a camera, microphone, and the Internet. Some web-conferencing systems even allow for break-out rooms in which students can meet separately in smaller groups and then come back to the entire class and share the highlights of their group work. Student presentations are also an activity that may be maximized via web conferencing, although if the classes are large, it may be better to have the students record their presentations and post them for viewing prior to the web-conferencing session. In that way, the time together as a class can be used to discuss and critique what has already been viewed.

Clarifying the Blended Format for Students

While it may be apparent to faculty why a course is considered "blended," it cannot be assumed that students will have a clear understanding. It should be explicitly stated at the start of the course in a "welcome" announcement that the course is blended and what delivery formats will be used. The purpose of the different delivery formats should be explained to students to help them understand how and why these formats are important to the learning process. A general statement might be used in the welcome statement, such as: "The blended format is designed to give students the opportunity to combine the convenience of online coursework with more real-time, individualized attention that meets a variety of learning styles. In-class and web-conferencing sessions allow students to participate in face-to-face interactive contact with instructors and peers." Students will also need to know where to find the delivery components of the course, when and where they should participate each week, and a structured set of topics and schedule for each specifying the dates, times, and locations of synchronous meetings.

Clarification of course delivery methods might be made by creating separate modules for in-class, online, and web-conferencing sessions. Then, in the introduction to each module, the course delivery format could be highlighted with a rationale as to why that particular format is being used to cover selected content. Separate modules for in-class and web-conferencing sessions might also be included with specific objectives for those sessions as well as directions on how to prepare for the sessions with requirements for participation. For other courses that may have online and clinical delivery components, modules may be used to cover the information to be delivered online, and a separate section created in the course management system detailing the information and schedule related to the clinical aspect of the course.

CONNECTING LEARNING ACTIVITIES ACROSS DELIVERY FORMATS

Although the delivery format for particular learning activities should be clear to the students, the connections among them across formats should also be obvious. For example, faculty might initially assign readings, short videos, or taped lectures as an introduction to content, and make these available to students asynchronously online. These kinds of activities might be followed by an interactive web-conferencing session with the purpose of having the students engage in a discussion of the material they previously reviewed with a set of structured questions. Sequencing these activities within the same learning module on a specific theme clarifies the relationship between the activities, and acknowledges their mutual reinforcement of each other.

Another example of connecting activities across delivery formats occurs with faculty and student introductions. If the course begins with a classroom-based session, introductions of faculty and students can easily be incorporated into the class activities. Introductions serve a number of purposes. They are the first step in developing relationships among the faculty and students to build a community of learning, and they create a sense of connection. Faculty introductions also are an opportunity to share one's background and expertise, philosophy of learning, role in the course, and experience in teaching blended courses. The introduction should also be delivered in a manner that encourages approachability.

Even if introductions are begun in a live interactive session, best practices support repeating them online in blended courses. This repetition not only serves as a reminder to students who may have forgotten what was said during the initial session, but also is available to students who may have missed the session. The online introduction may include all that was shared in the real-time session as well as a picture, email address, phone number, and best days and times to be reached by phone or email. With the increase in diversity of cultures of students, the introduction should include the instructor's preference on how he or she wishes to be addressed. It is up to the faculty member whether to also include personal information such as family and interests outside of his or her professional life. However, many instructors feel as if sharing some personal information increases the sense of social presence, or helps them be seen as real persons rather than objects, and contributes toward becoming more approachable by students.

Student introductions are also extremely helpful in building the learning community and making those connections. Students can learn much from their peers if they comfortable interacting with them. Again, even if students have an opportunity to introduce themselves during an initial live session, it should also be available online for future reference. Clear instructions on what to include in the introduction should be given, and students should be encouraged to share some personal information. It is often this kind of information that helps other students gravitate toward someone who shares their same background or interests and helps them begin to build a personal connection.

ADVANTAGES AND DISADVANTAGES
OF A BLENDED LEARNING

The number one advantage of the blended approach is that it empowers the faculty and the student to utilize all available avenues for both teaching and learning. The delivery of the teaching can take on many different formats and use multiple technologies to achieve a single objective. McCown (2010) summarizes the advantages of blended learning into the following areas for both faculty and students: flexibility, convenience, thoughtful participation, ability to use electronic tools and the Internet, and independent learning. Instructors have the flexibility to choose an instructional method and modality that best fits their teaching style, the content to be covered, and the targeted objective. This same flexibility transfers to students. Students with different learning styles are given the opportunity to gravitate toward the methods that best reaches them. These opportunities can be seen in the chosen delivery of the content, the flexibility of when and where to consume the content, and the possibilities of how to complete an assignment. It is noteworthy that student satisfaction and performance can be predicated on course design, delivery, and an environment that permits students to communicate with not only the faculty, but also with each other (Babb, Stewart, & Johnson, 2010). The core components of good course design need to be applied to and emphasized with the blended model, as they are sometimes overshadowed by the sheer complexity of the design.

Although most traditional face-to-face courses are able to meet the needs of students who fall within the middle of the bell curve in relation to meeting the learning objectives of the course, some students need a different approach to be successful. A blended-learning approach allows the instructor to offer more occasions for students who may need remediation to be successful in gaining a deeper understanding of content. It may also provide more flexibility in offering opportunities for students to pursue their interests well beyond the required objectives of the course. This flexibility also gives seasoned students more opportunities in a variety of formats to be successful and get the most out of their educational experience.

Although the flexibility available through a blended-learning approach may be seen as a significant advantage, it can also become a disadvantage in that the complexity of learning modes can be overwhelming for some faculty and students. If a faculty member or student has not previously experienced a blended course or program, it may be difficult to grasp the individual components and how they fit together. Therefore, it is important for both groups to have a strong orientation to the blended approach including how it relates to their role. The orientation should start with the whole picture view to ensure understanding of the entire system, and then focus on the components of the system.

There can also be a lack of flexibility if the instructor has to quickly move content from one format to another. Because so much planning goes into having the different delivery modes "fit" together, when an event requires an immediate change in delivery format, the process can have a snowball effect. For example, a face-to-face, classroom-based session may have to be abruptly canceled due to bad weather, or a technical problem causes a web-conferencing session to crash. Because these delivery modes were most likely selected as the best format for meeting specific learning objectives or delivering particular exercises and activities, having to accommodate a last-minute change can be formidable. Often, synchronous sessions are planned months in advance with guest speakers and pre-scheduled space. Rescheduling the session may be highly problematic or impossible. At the last minute the instructor may have to revise the entire lesson plan into an asynchronous format.

Another disadvantage relates to the technical context within which the student and faculty are consuming the technology-delivered material. While most academic settings post minimum technical specifications on admission, and all content should be created with those specifications in mind, access to the Internet is not always a known variable or a controllable one. Crawford and McKenzie (2011) ascertain that the ways in which students experience e-learning techniques are strongly influenced by Internet connectivity and broadband levels.

Blended learning offers advantages and disadvantages to students who enroll with disabilities. Madaus, Banerjee, McKeown, and Gelbar (2011) found that blended courses can provide both new opportunities and advantages for students with learning disabilities and Attention Deficit/Hyperactivity Disorder (ADHD), but at the same time brings the difficulties of the classroom and online environment with them. For example, the online mode of delivery may be more convenient and accessible for students with mobility impairments. In contrast, students with learning disabilities or other less visible disabilities (e.g., ADHD) may be less likely to self-disclose their disability and seek accommodations. More information on the issues and strategies related to online learning and students with learning disabilities can be found at LD Online (www.ldonline.org/) and the University of Connecticut, Center on Postsecondary Education and Disability (www.udi.uconn.edu/index.php?q=content/technical-brief-students-disabilities-and-online-learning).

FACULTY AND COURSE EVALUATIONS
IN A BLENDED COURSE

A strong evaluation plan is essential for faculty to improve their courses, as well as enhance and ensure quality education for students. The evaluation strategies should be designed to elicit feedback on all aspects of the blended course. The purpose is to obtain student perceptions about the instructional strategies, learning activities/resources, technological aspects of the course, and course delivery formats. However, the evaluation strategies for a blended course should be less focused on the technology and mode of course delivery, and should explore the effectiveness of the delivery format for achieving the learning objectives. For example, a 5-point Likert scale ranging from Strongly Disagree to Strongly Agree might be used for evaluation purposes, and includes statements such as:

▦ The amount of contact with the instructor has met my needs.
▦ The balance of course delivery formats facilitated meeting the course objectives.
▦ Working on group assignments with my peers via web conferencing has contributed to a sense of a learning community.

Periodic assessments can be scheduled during the in-class and web-conferencing sessions in which discussions or interactive exercises may serve as opportunities for a formative evaluation of students' understanding of the content presented online. Mid-semester evaluations can be very useful in identifying strengths and weaknesses in the course, which can allow for immediate improvements to the course. End-of-course summative evaluations of blended courses offer students a means to provide input for assessing and improving course design, course delivery, and teaching performance. Through anonymous end-of-semester course evaluations, students give instructors and the university feedback about the effectiveness, quality, and value of courses. This feedback often plays an important role in course improvement as well as faculty review processes.

Faculty teaching blended courses benefit from using established benchmarks when designing and evaluating their courses (Babb, 2010). The *Quality Matters Program* (2011–2013) has received national recognition for developing a research-based rubric consisting of 8 general standards and 41 specific criteria that describe best practices in online and blended learning. The rubric is used as part of a collaborative peer review process with the primary aim of ensuring quality assurance and continuous improvement. The rubric includes annotations that are focused specifically on blended courses, and provides recommendations for how to handle introductions, scheduling, explanations of purposes of delivery formats, and connections/sequencing among the course delivery modes. Other similar tools are available for the design and evaluation of online courses, such as the California State University (Chico) Rubric for Online Instruction (2009) and Illinois Online Network (2008) online course initiative rubric, which can also be used to evaluate blended courses with significant online components.

REFERENCES

Ackerman, A. S. (2008a). Blended learning ingredients: A cooking metaphor. *Journal of Instruction Delivery Systems, 22*(3), 21–25.

Ackerman, A. S. (2008b). Hybrid learning in higher education: Engagement strategies. *Media Review, 14*(1), 145–158.

Adelman, D. S. & Nogueras, D. J. (2013). Discussion boards: Boring no more! *Nurse Educator, 38*(1), 30–33.

Allen, L. A., Seaman, J., & Garrett, R. (2007). *Blending in: The extent and promise of blended education in the United States.* Needham, MA: Sloan Consortium. Retrieved from http://sloanconsortium.org/publications/survey/pdf/Blending_In.pdf

Babb, S., Stewart, C., & Johnson, R. (2010). Constructing communication in blended learning environments: Students' perceptions of good practice in hybrid courses. *Journal of Online Learning and Teaching, 6*(4). Retrieved from http://jolt.merlot.org/vol6no4/babb_1210.htm

California State University at Chico. (2009). *Rubric for online instruction.* Retrieved from http://www.csuchico.edu/tlp/resources/rubric/rubric.pdf

Crawford, N., & McKenzie, L. E. (2011). Learning in context: An assessment of student inequalities in a university outreach program. *Australasian Journal of Educational Technology, 27*(3), 531–545.

Illinois Online Network and the Board of Trustees of the University of Illinois. (2008). *A tool to assist in the design, redesign, and/or evaluation of online courses.* Retrieved from http://www.icc.edu/innovation/forms/QOCIReformat.pdf

Madaus, J. W., Banerjee, M., McKeown, K., & Gelbar, N. (2011). Online and blended learning: The advantages and the challenges for students with learning disabilities and attention deficit/hyperactivity disorder. *Learning Disabilities: A Multidisciplinary Journal, 17*(2), 69–76.

McCown, L. (2010). Blended courses: The best of online and traditional formats. *Clinical Laboratory Science, 23*(4), 205–211.

Palloff, R., & Pratt, K. (2007). *Building online learning communities: Effective strategies for the virtual classroom.* San Francisco: Jossey-Bass.

Quality Matters Program. (2011–2013). *Quality matters rubric standards 2011–2013 edition with assigned point values.* Retrieved from http://www .qmprogram.org/files/QM_Standards_2011-2013.pdf

Rovai, A. P., & Jordan, H. M. (2004). Blended learning and sense of community: A comparative analysis with traditional and fully online graduate courses. *International Review of Research in Open and Distance Learning, 5*(2). Retrieved from http://www.irrodl.org/index.php/irrodl/article/view/192/274

Short, J., Williams, E., & Christie, B. (1976). *The social psychology of telecommunications.* London: John Wiley & Sons.

Staker, H., Horn, M. B., & Innosight, I. (2012). Classifying K-12 blended learning. *Innosight Institute.* Retrieved from http://www.innosightinstitute .org/innosight/wp-content/uploads/2012/05/Classifying-K-12-blended-learning2.pdf

Watson, J. (2008). *Blended learning: The convergence of online and face-to-face education. Promising practices in online learning.* Vienna, VA: North American Council for Online Learning. Retrieved from http://www.eric. ed.gov/PDFS/ED509636.pdf

Watson, J. & Gemin, B. (2010). *The state of online learning in Maryland.* Retrieved from http://www.marylandpublicschools.org/NR/rdonlyres/D895AEF0-476A-46CF-86E5-A77C87A4E129/27450/OnlineLearning_MD_2010_2011.pdf

EIGHT

Interacting and Communicating Online

CHERYL A. FISHER

Instructional interactivity takes place among the instructor, the learners, and the content (Figure 8.1), and each interaction must be considered in the instructional design. In a traditional classroom, communication between the teacher and the student and among students is generally synchronous (occurring at the same time and place). In distance learning, communication can be either synchronous or asynchronous (not occurring at the same time). When faculty and students interact and engage in the face-to-face classroom, they develop intellectual and personal bonds. The same type of bonding happens in an online setting (Boettcher, 2011). This chapter discusses different types of interaction and communication that are well suited for distance courses.

IMPORTANCE OF INTERACTION

A successful online course is easy to access, easy to navigate, and makes it easy to interact with others. Interactivity means more than just clicking a mouse button to advance to the next page. Interactivity requires meaningful feedback (i.e., leading toward an established goal) for each learner. Purposes for providing online discussion might

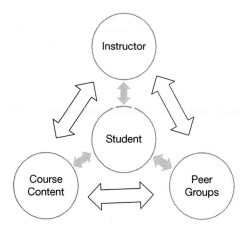

FIGURE 8.1   Elements of interaction in online learning environments.

include: to provide an open question-and-answer forum, to encourage critical thinking, to achieve social interaction and community building, to validate experiences, and to support student reflections and inquiries (Grogan, 2005). Often this involves written confirmation of a correct response, or a dialogue with the instructor or other learners. In the online environment, interaction can take place in the form of a question-and-answer session, an essay, or a discussion, and may be asynchronous or synchronous. Moore (1993) described three types of interaction that are critical to student learning in the online environment: 1) learner to content, 2) learner to instructor, and 3) learner to learner. Learner-to-learner interaction is important as it can take place in the form of group activities or group discussion forums (Figure 8.1)

The characteristics of a "good" online conversation include evidence of problem solving, informed decision making, and depth of both student and teacher facilitated discussions. There should also be evidence of episodes that extend the conversation beyond a simple question-and-answer interaction to the examination of complex problems from multiple perspectives. The environment should be designed to facilitate and promote critical thinking, knowledge expansion and opportunities for students to draw from their experiences. Questions that encourage exploration and research might include Socratic-type probing, such as:

Why do you think that?
What is your reasoning?

Is there an alternative strategy?
From your experiences, did you find this to be the case?
Can you expand on what you mentioned in your post?

The online environment can be structured for effective social constructivist learning utilizing interactive online discussion and Socratic questioning. These models of collaborative learning are becoming mandatory in course design and delivery as online learning is incorporated into institutional policies.

Flottemesch (2000) noted in a literature review that students tend to judge the quality of distance-based education on their perceived interaction in the course. Giguere, Formica, and Harding (2004), who studied interaction and professional development, found that interaction had less to do with personal interaction (e.g., building a community of learners) and more to do with providing a means of reinforcing various elements from the content of the training. Other research suggests that learning in groups improves students' achievement of learning objectives and in some cases grades (Chiong & Jovanovick, 2012). Little investigation, however, has been done to compare the effects of different types of interaction (peer to peer, student to instructor) on learning in distance learning environments.

ASYNCHRONOUS COMMUNICATION

Asynchronous communication means that communication occurs at different times. It is characterized by time independence, meaning the sender and receiver communicate with time delays. When preparing online courses, instructors build mechanisms into the instructional design for asynchronous communication such as email, electronic bulletin boards, discussion boards, or wikis. Email allows for personal, private communication and direct feedback. The electronic bulletin board is used for all participants to post and read messages. This form of asynchronous communication is most commonly used in main discussion areas of online classrooms or the web and allows students to interact with faculty, other students, and course content.

Instructor-to-Student Interactions

It is suggested that instructor and student interaction is one of the most critical factors in distance learning outcomes (Pallof & Pratt,

2001; Salmon, 2001; Shea, 2011). Due to the physical separation of learners and instructors, technology plays a vital role in providing a learning experience compatible with a face-to-face course. Shur (2011) further states that interactions are significant contributors to the level of student learning and satisfaction and are consistent with learning theories that emphasize the importance of the learning process. In a review of the literature by Meyer (2002), she noted that quality learning is largely the result of ample interaction with the faculty, other students, and content.

Student-to-Content Interactions

In traditional environments, textbooks, PowerPoint® slide shows, and video clips compose the instructional content for a class. In distance courses, instructors can decide how best to deliver course content along with the guidance of an instructional designer. More sophisticated delivery modes are becoming popular as increased bandwidth and fiber optics allow for the downloading of multimedia files, PowerPoint, Flash®, or YouTube® presentations (with or without associated audio), and streaming video. However, the instructor should not convert materials used in traditional courses without considering how distance technologies allow the course materials to be used more effectively and efficiently. Additionally, the instructor needs to consider whether the students are able to access multimedia requiring plug-ins for viewing and to access large data files. Because some students may still access the Internet using dialup modems, the time required to download large files should be supplemented with a smaller file option (i.e., a text version of an audio file). This will allow the students to have options for accessing course information based on preference and bandwidth capability.

Depending on how the technology is used, students may find it easier to use or interact with distance learning content than with traditional classroom content. Instructor notes or slides available for print from the course site allow students to take notes more thoroughly while listening to online lectures. Graphics or animated images available online can be viewed over and over by students without having to go to the library or nursing lab. Animated graphics create simulations to demonstrate blood flow or actions of the cranial nerves and help students visualize body processes better than a one-dimensional textbook is capable of showing. An example of one of these automations can be viewed at www.nobelprize.org/educational/medicine/immunity/ where gaming is used to teach specifics related to immunology, blood typing, and other topics. Another example can be found at www.wilkes.med.ucla.edu/inex.htm where students can learn about heart sounds and murmurs through descriptive and auditory methodologies.

Student-to-Student Interactions

Student-to-student interaction using asynchronous communication can take place in the main discussion area of an online course or in collaborative groups. The main discussion area of an online course should be analogous to the main classroom in a face-to-face course. This discussion area is where the students and the instructor should meet to participate in active dialogue and discuss course material. It is also where students have the opportunity to learn from each other and ask questions for further understanding of course content. It is this interaction that is an important component of the learning dynamic and it is technology that is responsible for bringing students together. Because effective use of the discussion board requires some extra effort, the result is actually more interaction (Gilbert, 2001). Since students cannot hide in an online course, especially when drawn into interaction by the instructor, the result is active participation that is often not observed in a face-to-face classroom. Students often feel less inhibited and have time to collect their thoughts prior to speaking up in an asynchronous discussion.

Group Collaboration

Groups or learning teams are another means by which the instructor can promote collaboration and interaction in the online classroom. Creating teams is useful for the purpose of small group discussion, completion of group assignments, engagement in small group activities, and simulations (Palloff & Pratt, 1999). When there is a variety of activities and experiences, online course work can be more enjoyable and effective. This allows students to work through concepts, brainstorm, and work together. Building in options and opportunities for students to work together or individually is also highly recommended (Boettcher, 2011). Groups or teams can be especially effective when working on case scenarios or problem-based learning (PBL) activities.

Teams can be formed by offering students the opportunity to self-select membership or by instructor assignment. Sometimes students like to work together based on past experience and sometimes by time zones. Once groups are formed, it is important to post guidelines and expectations of team performance. For example:

1. Each team will designate, elect, or appoint a team coordinator or leader.
2. The leader will remain the same throughout the course unless replaced by a majority vote of the team or by the instructor.
3. The team leader may make a decision unless overruled by a majority.
4. Any project assigned to the group will receive a grade that applies to every member of that group.
5. The team leader will have the opportunity for input regarding any team member's grade.
6. The instructor will have the final say in all cases where the team cannot reach a decision.

Within these guidelines it is expected that the team members will evaluate each other's work, participate, and contribute to the team assignment. Team self-evaluation is an option to offer teams to help promote a productive work environment. For example, the instructor might ask: 1) What worked, 2) what needed improvement, and 3) how would you make these improvements?

Synchronous Communication

Synchronous communication can take place in the form of Skype or interactive videoconferencing. The greatest challenge of synchronous communication or meetings is to coordinate a time when all participants are available. Considerations that need to be made are differences in time zones, students working different shifts, and the hardware requirements (i.e., web cam).

The logistics of timing live meetings can truly be reason enough not to use them. If students are working shifts in different time zones, it may be impossible to find a time that is convenient for all. Nurses working the night shift may have to get up in the middle of the day to participate. This will lead to reduced quality in their contributions and disruption in sleep prior to going back to work. When students are dispersed internationally, the window for meeting times is further reduced.

In the online environment, Internet meetings using web cameras can be used, but this technology currently works best for a small number of individuals. Synchronous video conferencing or webinars require students to be at a certain place at a certain time; it is beginning to be used more in graduate-level courses. Possibilities for actual participation in lectures offered in remote places exist, but may require that the student visit a campus that has the video conferencing technology in place. This technology allows students in several locations to share the same learning experience simultaneously through two-way video and audio.

BUILDING COMMUNITY

Regardless of whether you use asynchronous or synchronous communication in the online classroom, students should feel as if they are a part of the learning community. Distance students often feel isolated and alone in their early experiences online, but with proper guidance and personalized attention, they quickly bond and come to depend on each other for learning and moral support. It is the instructor's responsibility to facilitate the personal and social aspects of an online community in order to create a successful learning experience (Palloff & Pratt, 1999). Collins and Berge (1996) write that promoting human relationships by affirming and recognizing students' input, providing opportunities for students to develop a sense of group cohesiveness, maintaining the group as a unit, and helping members to work together for a mutual goal are necessary elements for building community in an online environment.

So how does an instructor begin to develop a sense of community in an online course? Many begin with introductions or an initial request for posting of a biography. The instructor can model how the "bio" is to be posted by posting one first and asking for 1) professional experiences, 2) educational background, and 3) personal information. The bios will allow students to find commonalities and provide the opportunity to get to know each other. Another technique may be to use ice breakers. Online ice breakers can include games or strategies to get students to talk about themselves; for example, "the ABCs of me" or "post eight nouns about yourself." These ice breakers allow students to seek others in the class with similar interests or experiences that may facilitate good working relationships. Another strategy for facilitating community is to set up an area called cyber chat or a student lounge where students can meet and greet without loading up the main classroom with personal chatter.

New generations of social software show a human face online and help students and faculty communicate, educate, and interact with their communities. These new software tools include blogs, wikis, social networking software, photo sharing, podcasting, and more. The ease of use and popularity of these new communication methodologies have potential for tremendous impact and are making up what is being described as Web 2.0 technologies. However, as some students may not be familiar with these new technologies it is going to require alignment of the task and the technology in order for the benefit to be realized and the integration to be seamless.

ACTIVE LEARNING

In order to actively engage learners in the online learning process and to facilitate the meaning-making process that is a part of the constructivist approach through which this learning occurs, the content of the course should be embedded in everyday life (Palloff & Pratt, 1999). In other words, the more learners can relate their life experience and what they already know to the context of the online classroom, the deeper their understanding will be of what they learn. In nursing, for example, students should be provided with case-based scenarios or problems to resolve based on their area of interest in nursing.

The online instructor can promote active learning through the creative use of instructional design strategies. For example, the incorporation of web quests or PBL scenarios will facilitate meaningful active learning and help students search for real-life answers. A web quest is an inquiry-oriented activity in which some or all of the information that learners interact with comes from resources on the Internet (Dodge, 1997). Web quests can be of either short or long duration and are deliberately designed to make the best use of a learner's time. Web quests should contain at least the following components:

- An introduction that sets the stage and provides some background information.
- A task that is doable and interesting.

- A set of information sources needed to complete the task. Many (though not necessarily all) of the resources are embedded in the web quest document itself as anchors pointing to information on the web. Information sources might include web documents, experts who are available via email or real-time conferencing, searchable databases on the net, and books and other documents physically available in the learner's setting. Because pointers to resources are included, the learner is not left to wander through web space completely adrift.
- A description of the process the learners should go through in accomplishing the task. The process should be broken down into clearly described steps.
- Some guidance on how to organize the information acquired. This may take the form of guiding questions or directions to complete organizational frameworks such as timelines, concept maps, or cause-and-effect diagrams.
- A conclusion that brings closure to the quest, reminds the learners about what they've learned, and perhaps encourages them to extend the experience into other domains.

Several examples of nursing web quests are available on the web. One example is a web quest that provides nursing students with an activity related to describing the role of the professional nurse (see edtech2.boisestate.edu/loefflerd/edtech512/Modules/Webquest512/intro.html). This web quest seeks to promote a discussion about the role of professional nursing and to help students develop a clear understanding of what professional nursing is. Another example can be found at zunal.com/stats.php?w=102162, which was developed for graduate students to help them provide compassionate care at the end of life. Free software for developing similar creative learning opportunities is available at www. Zunal.com.

PBL using case-based scenarios are another example of active learning strategies that can be used by instructors to promote collaboration among teams of students. As described in Chapter 2, PBL is an instructional method that challenges students to "learn to learn," working cooperatively in groups to seek solutions to real-world problems. These problems are used to engage students' curiosity and initiate learning the subject matter. PBL prepares students to think critically and analytically, and to find and use appropriate learning resources. With its roots in the medical profession, PBL was originally developed to assist interns to determine a diagnosis based on the given symptoms of a patient. PBL promotes student initiative as a driving force and supports a system of student–faculty interaction in which the student assumes primary responsibility for the process (Neville, 2009).

Cognitive apprenticeship is another strategy that involves close communication between experts and novices in an authentic context. Nurses taking clinical courses in community health, adult health, or other practical areas will need to be involved in this type of learning experience. In this environment, novices progress along a path to expertise by refining authentic products and processes under the mentorship of experts. Cognitive apprenticeships are situated within the social constructivist paradigm and suggest that students work in teams on projects or problems. They are representative of Vygotski's "zones of proximal development" in which student tasks are slightly more difficult than students can manage independently, requiring the aid of their peers and instructor to succeed (Brown, Collins, & Duguid,1989).

As with any apprenticeship, this involves observation of experts in action, coaching of novices by experts, and successive approximation to expert work as novices gain expertise. The students may be physically present in a hospital or community to develop skills while participating in the didactic part of the course online. Ongoing dialogue and conversations between and among students and instructors will help students to identify problems that they may encounter or skills that they need to develop.

In summary, interaction and communication has been identified as the core of the course where learning takes place in an online environment. It is the interaction among instructors, students, and the course content that is necessary in order for the content to be applied and knowledge to be developed. Group activities and active learning techniques should be applied and are characteristic of a constructivist learning environment. Web quests, PBL, and cognitive apprenticeships are examples of active learning strategies that are well suited to the online classroom and work well with online nursing courses.

REFERENCES

Boettcher, J. (2011). Ten best practices for teaching online: Quick guide for new online faculty. Retrieved January 30, 2013, from http://www .designingforlearning.info/services/writing/ecoach/tenbest.html

Brown, J. S., Collins, A., & Duguid, P. (1989). Situated cognition and the culture of learning. *Educational Researcher, 18*, 32–42.

Chiong, R., & Jovanovic, J. (2012). Collaborative learning in online study groups: An evolutionary game theory perspective. *Journal of Education Technology: Research, 11.*

Collins, M., & Berge. Z. (1996). Facilitating interaction in computer mediated online courses. Retrieved April 3, 2008, from http://www.emoderators.com/moderators/flcc.html

Dodge, B. (1997). Web quests: A technique for internet-based learning. *Distance Educator, 1*(2), 10–13.

Flottemesch, K. (2000). Building effective interaction in distance education: A review of the literature. *Educational Technology, 40*(3), 46–51.

Giguere, P., Formica, S., & Harding, W. (2004). Large scale interaction strategies for web-based professional development. *American Journal of Distance Education, 18*(4), 207–223.

Gilbert, S. D. (2001). *How to be a successful online student.* New York, NY: McGraw Hill Professional.

Grogan, G. (2005). *The design of online discussions to achieve good learning results.* Retrieved January 30, 2013, from www.elearningeuropa.info/index .php?page=doc&doc_id=6713&doclng=6&menuzone=1

Meyer, K. (2002). Quality in distance education: Focus on online learning. In A. J. Kezar (Ed.), *ASHE-ERIC higher education report,* (pp. i–vii). San Francisco, CA: Jossey-Bass.

Moore, M. (1993). Transactional distance theory. In D. Keegan. (Ed.), *Theoretical Principles of Distance Education.* New York, NY: Routledge.

Neville, A. J. (2009). Problem-based learning and medical education forty years on. A review of its effects on knowledge and clinical performance. *Medical Principles and Practice. 18*(1):1–9.

Palloff, R. & Pratt, K. (1999). *Building learning communities in cyberspace: Effective strategies for the online classroom.* SanFrancisco: JosseyBass.

NINE

Course Management Methods

CHERYL A. FISHER

Many instructors, due to their academic setting, are expected to deliver high quality instruction to people who would otherwise not be able to participate in higher education. This presents an exciting and challenging opportunity for collaborative learning and is affecting the way traditional classes are taught. In 2013, 6.7 million students participated in distance learning and nearly one third of all students are taking at least one online course (Going the Distance, Online Education in the United States). Managing an online course can have many similarities to managing a face-to-face course but will differ in complexity with the use of technology, new Web 2.0 technology, geography, and the many new technologies becoming available. However, it is through the use of this rapid expansion and application of technology that the online learning environment is becoming a richer and sometimes preferred place to learn.

Facilitating learning at a distance requires faculty to take some new approaches to managing the teaching and learning process. The faculty role in the online classroom requires greater attention to detail, structure, and monitoring of student activity. According to Vitale (2010), effective online faculty are becoming critical in order to deal with the nursing shortage and faculty must learn to manage a new set of variables that determines the extent to which their courses are effective. In this chapter, the role of the instructor in planning, organizing, and managing the online learning environment, along with the expectations of the student, are discussed.

FACULTY ROLE

The role of the instructor shifts from the traditional classroom "sage on the stage" to the "guide on the side." Although these might be overused phrases, there is a lot of truth to them when applied to the instructor role shift that takes place when teaching online. In addition to technological and pedagogical changes, research substantiates that the evolving distance learning phenomenon has an impact on the role of faculty (Ryan, Hodson-Carlton, & Ali, 2005). In a traditional setting, the instructor feeds information to students in a lecture or PowerPoint® slide presentation format, creating a teacher-centered environment. This method of teaching has long been used in educational settings and has come to be what most students expect. In a distance learning role, the instructor focuses on discussing and reviewing materials presented through video and audio technologies, assigned readings, and interactive group activities. The faculty role is that of content expert who guides or facilitates student learning through direction to resources and stimulation of discussion, thereby creating a student-centered environment. A trained facilitator is important to the success of an online program and the prospects can be overwhelming to faculty new to online teaching. The facilitator's training, personality, professionalism, and knowledge of the content become important factors influencing the online classroom.

Faculty training for teaching online may differ significantly from face-to-face instruction. Currently there is no single approach and many institutions are using a combination of training and mentoring. Ninety-four percent of institutions with online offerings report that they have training or mentoring programs for their online faculty (Going the Distance, www.onlinelearningsurvey.com/reports/goingthedistance.pdf). The most common training approaches for online faculty are internally run training and informal mentoring. Some smaller institutions report looking to outside institutions for their training needs.

According to the Illinois Online Network (ION), the responsibilities and pressures on instructors require faculty to look at teaching students in a new way. Some feel the pressure of a classroom that is open 24 hours a day with adult learners who might require additional support due to their already busy lives. Some responsibilities include:

- Planning and organizing the course
- Creating a collaborative atmosphere
- Providing opportunities for teamwork
- Constructing open-ended, thought-provoking questions
- Providing direction and leadership
- Setting the agenda
- Formative and summative evaluation

In order to perform these responsibilities, successful online faculty should have some basic background knowledge and preparation to teach online. The ION (2013) identifies that the online instructor should have a broad base of life experiences in addition to academic credentials in the subject matter. This will enable the instructor to actively participate with students and guide their constructive thinking. Other skills required to be successful include:

- Be open, concerned, flexible, and sincere so one can compensate for the lack of physical presence.
- Feel comfortable communicating in writing.
- Believe that learning can occur in facilitated online learning environments.
- Believe that the online learning process includes learning information that can be used today and that requires critical thinking.
- Be supportive of the development of critical thinking.
- Have the appropriate credentials to teach the subject.
- Be well trained in teaching and learning online.

Teaching in a technology-rich environment is complex and therefore requires a broader set of skills and competencies from the faculty facilitators in order to ensure success. A study conducted by Gigatel, Ragan, Kennan, May, and Redmond (2012) identified competencies and teaching tasks aimed at providing faculty with professional development in critical competencies to ensure online teaching success. These competencies focused on the areas of active learning and engaging with students as appropriate, administration and leadership, active teaching and providing prompt helpful feedback, use of multimedia appropriate for learning activities, classroom decorum to help students resolve potential conflicts, technological competence, and policy enforcement. These competencies closely mirror but expand on the seven principles of effective teaching identified by Chickering and Ehrman in 1996.

PLANNING AND ORGANIZING

When planning and organizing an online course, the instructor must look at the overall course in terms of objectives, outcomes, assessment, and evaluation. The planning should include the criteria discussed in the reconceptualization chapter of this book (Chapter 5). The instructor should keep in mind that it is in this beginning phase of course development that an instructional designer and an information technology expert should be consulted for best practices.

The curriculum of an online program must be designed especially for the collaborative nature of online learning. Course content should be organized in modules with clear deadlines for the assigned work in each section. These concise lectures should be compensated with open-ended remarks and discussion questions that will elicit comments and provide the students' opportunities to contribute a variety of viewpoints. The curriculum should focus on applying knowledge utilizing real-world examples and fostering critical thinking skills within the opportunities of exchanging ideas. Instructors should give clear and simple assignments with clear instructions.

COLLABORATION

Once the course has been planned and organized, the instructor is ready to launch the course. It is now the instructor's responsibility to create a collaborative atmosphere. To create this environment, the students should encounter a friendly, welcoming message as they first enter the online course. Using an "ice breaker" such as requesting a short biography and a photo as the initial assignment will give students something to which they can respond. The instructor can post his or her bio as an introduction and then ask the students to present theirs in a similar format. This is not only a way of introducing oneself to the class but also a way for the instructor to gain information about students that can be used later in class discussions. The students often find that they have similar backgrounds or professional interests, which then allows them to begin developing a sense of community through realization of shared goals and shared expectations of the course. By asking the learners to contribute their goals and expectations, the instructor is able to determine if his or her approach to the course will correspond more closely to the needs of the learners.

Students should be encouraged to respond to each other's postings. The best way to teach students how to post meaningful statements is for the instructor to model how they should respond. Modeling a short but welcoming response does this best. Not only does this enable students to begin opening up to each other, but it begins to create a safe space in which they can interact. The posting of an introduction is the first step in revealing who one is to the others in the class, and it is critical that students feel acknowledged so they can continue to do that safely throughout the duration of the course. This is the first point of connection—the point where these important relationships begin to develop (Palloff & Pratt, 1999).

DEVELOPING DISCUSSION QUESTIONS

Developing or creating open-ended questions is the primary method for stimulating discussion, assessing student learning, and providing for interactivity among the learners. More and more evidence is emerging about the value of interaction between faculty and students to promote effective teaching. The discussion questions should be based on the desired learning outcomes and can vary in number based on instructor preference. The discussion questions should be open ended, thought provoking, and relevant to student learning. Then, the instructor as well as the students must learn the art of expansive questions in order to keep the discussion going. This allows the responsibility for facilitation of discussion to be shared among all participants. And finally, students should be encouraged to provide constructive feedback to one another throughout the course. Rather than being at the forefront of the discussion, the instructor is an equal player, acting as a gentle guide (Palloff & Pratt, 1999). The sharing of this responsibility among the participants is one way instructors can stretch their facilitative skills.

The discussion questions should be developed in such a way that there is no right or wrong answer. They serve to stimulate thinking and are a means by which the instructor can assess student learning and understanding of the issues. The instructor needs to model this form of questioning so that students can learn to answer questions in a substantive manner, provide an example, cite a resource, and end with an expansive question of their own for their peers. This allows for the discussion to progress to a higher level as questions are answered and expanded upon by students pursuing the issue. The instructor's role is to closely monitor the discussion and to jump in with another question, thereby expanding the level of thinking beyond the original question. A poor or minimal response to a question could indicate that student thinking has not been stimulated and that the learners have not been compelled or inspired to respond. Commenting on discussion questions by asking students for more information or by sharing some aspects of their professional expertise can help to engage students and facilitate online discussions.

Some examples of the behaviors that faculty must exhibit to meet the competency of active learning include encouraging student interactivity by assigning them to team projects and groups for project purposes, encouraging shared knowledge by providing opportunities for hands-on practice so that students can apply learned knowledge to the real world; for example, with problem solving activities and peer-to-peer assessment. These tasks can promote active learning and are skills required by faculty to promote learning.

DIRECTION AND LEADERSHIP

Providing direction and leadership in an online course should begin before the students enter the classroom. The syllabus or a separate document on how to run the course provides clear directions for students about the following aspects of the course:

- General information
- Contact information

■ Textbooks or other course materials
■ Course requirements
■ Where to start
■ How I plan to run this course
■ Class schedule, parts of the classroom
■ Group work and expectations
■ Technical support
■ Grading
■ Student responsibility

General course information to include in the syllabus should include course start and end dates, project due dates, and midterm and final exam dates. Time off for spring break or other breaks related to holidays or official closing of the university should also be included on the course calendar. Contact information is important for students in order to have easy access to faculty. Often it is helpful to put a primary and a secondary email address, work and home phone numbers (optional), and the best times to make contact. Times of contact are important, especially when students are working shifts and faculty may be located in a different time zone. Required texts and supporting documents should be available to students before class begins or at least during the first week of class. Students should have the ability to order books from either the bookstore or another online book service such as Amazon. Other recommended texts should be listed in case students are interested in purchasing these as well.

Course requirements help students know in advance what they will need to do and what faculty has identified as requirements to complete this course; for example: view lecture material, complete assigned readings, participate in team exercises, complete assignments, and take midterm and final examinations. Listing requirements ahead of time will help students organize their approach to the course and will provide clarity of course requirements.

"Where to start" and "How I plan to run this course" documentation are opportunities to help students begin. In a face-to-face course, this is the housekeeping session that takes place on the first day of class. When directing students where to start, it is critical to have students attend either a face-to-face or an online orientation. It is in this orientation that they will be instructed to obtain a password for the course and begin to learn basic navigation of the courseware if this is their first experience with online learning. Once students are inside the online course, they should be directed to read the course information carefully. This should include the syllabus and all supporting documents that will be used to run the course.

The course schedule can be placed in a calendar and should include important dates that students should note. For example, weekly lectures and when discussion questions will be posted. This schedule will help students develop some structure for their learning and help them to juggle their workload. Let them know when quizzes will be posted, and again take the opportunity to highlight due dates of midterms, final exams, and papers. The instructor should make sure that students know how to access grades. One lesson for faculty that cannot be overstated is that you cannot be too redundant in the online environment. The more places a student can find important dates, the better. The main parts of the classroom should also be clearly delineated. If using courseware such as Blackboard or Moodle, the left menu bar is a good place to start designing the online classroom. For example:

Announcements: Frequent communications and important dates to remember should be posted here.

Course Information: This section should contain documents such as the syllabus, quizzes, sample of an American Psychological Association-formatted paper (or whatever style guide is required), instructions on submitting assignments and other pertinent documents.

Faculty Information: This section should contain contact information (as identified previously) as well as other information that might be useful while students are enrolled in your course.

Assignments: This section should contain instructions for individual assignments and the grading criteria.

Course Documents: This section houses course lectures, course objectives, readings, and supplemental web links for each lecture of the course. This is the primary location for the course content.

Student Tools: This is where the digital drop box, student grades, calendar, and other tools are located.

By identifying the parts of the online classroom, orientation information is restated and a text document is provided for reference. Once this document is written, it is highly reusable except for dates or changes that have taken place in the course. Technical support contact information should also be provided in the form of hours of availability, phone numbers, and email. Although this information is provided, invariably technical questions will show up in the discussion area of the classroom. Posting a message thread for technical questions will often allow students to answer each other's questions and keep the questions separate from the course content of the main classroom.

Grading information should also be clearly delineated in terms of: 1) methods of evaluation (i.e., class exercises, assignments, papers, rubrics, and exams), and 2) criteria for the final grade. For example:

Participation 10%
Team Exercises 30%
Midterm Exam 30%
Final Exam 30%
Total 100%

Just as in face-to-face classes, students need to know the weight of graded assignments. They should also know what percentage or point value is required for letter grades. This is also a good place to include the policy on late assignments (regarding point reduction) or incomplete grades, and information about the university's policy on academic integrity.

One aspect of ensuring quality and academic integrity is finding ways to document student identity as related to course assignments and testing. In short, faculty need to be sure that individuals receiving course credit are, indeed, the individuals who do the work. Institutions have a variety of ways to achieve identity security in the context of a meaningful assessment. The choices that an institution has will depend on the institutional resources, the type of assessment appropriate for measuring achievement of the learning objectives, and the number of students that need to be served. While high-tech methodologies exist for secure identification, such as retinal scanning or facial, voice, or fingerprint identification, institutions may not be ready to invest in these technologies. Another alternative is proctored testing centers or web-based testing software. This software requires a user name and password and can provide a different test each time the user logs in. Faculty should be familiar with the capabilities of the course management system or they can consult with technical support to determine best options.

SEQUENCE AND PACE

The sequence and pace of providing lectures and assignments can be left to the instructor's discretion. Some instructors prefer to post lectures, assignments, and discussion questions on a week-by-week basis. This controls the pace of the course and does not allow the students to work ahead. This model would most closely replicate the sequence and pace of a face-to-face classroom. Some instructors like to guide the online classroom discussion using this strategy. Another option would be to release course content by units or modules. Using this strategy, the instructor would still want to control the discussion by posting discussion questions regularly within the block of time designated for a particular unit. A third strategy for sequencing the release of course content would be to give the student the entire course at the beginning of class. Students will be required to participate according to the instructor's instructions. This strategy allows students to work ahead in their reading, writing, and group work, but also allows the instructor to control the collaborative learning in the main discussion area of the classroom. Some instructors have found it useful to put start and stop dates on discussions. For example, if a particular discussion thread is only going to be open for 2 weeks, the instructor should post start and stop dates at the beginning of the message thread so that students know when to move on to the next topic.

FEEDBACK

Feedback is one of the most critical activities that instructors need to be aware of in online learning because of the lack of face-to-face interaction. Feedback goes beyond confirmation of correct answers. Feedback is necessary for students to develop new understandings and to facilitate learning. Students need much more support and feedback in the online environment than in a traditional course in order to compensate for the lack of face-to-face interaction (ION, 2013). It is necessary for instructors to respond to students in a timely manner (usually within 24–48 hours) in order for students to feel encouraged to participate and to continue to participate at a high level. Online students need extra reinforcement and verification of their performance. Positive feedback, constructive feedback, and tone are all areas that instructors need to be aware of and sensitive to when responding to students. For example, proposing an alternative viewpoint might be interpreted by a student as an incorrect statement on the student's part as opposed to just an expansion of ideas. While maintaining a positive and encouraging tone and keeping things light with humor and emoticons (www.netlingo.com/smileys.php), the instructor can still maintain a professional atmosphere in the class environment.

Most instructors know that communicating with students can positively influence learning and can be done using feedback techniques. Because improvement in learning is more likely to occur following both written and oral critiques of student work, it is important to provide more than just a number or letter grade on student assignments. Written critiques or telephone conversations can be provided to students for more indepth explanations of grades, but more likely this will occur by email. The following characteristics should be considered in providing personal feedback to students:

■ Multidimensional (covers content, presentation, and grammar)
■ Nonevaluative (provides objective information)
■ Supportive (offers information that will allow the learner to see areas for improvement)
■ Receiver controlled (allows the learner to accept or reject the information)
■ Timely (provided as soon as possible after the intended work)
■ Specific (precisely describes observations and recommendations)

The instructor should be sure to provide information at the beginning of class so that students know what is expected of them and what will be standard for evaluation and feedback. Instructor feedback should be clear, thorough, consistent, equitable, and professional. Since students require regular and constructive feedback from faculty, they will appreciate comments that indicate the instructor has tailored remarks for that particular individual.

FORMATIVE AND SUMMATIVE FEEDBACK

As mentioned previously, gathering student feedback mid-course (formative) and at the end of the course (summative) are important for instructors to have the opportunity to make major or minor adjustments. Gathering feedback mid course should be short, anonymous, and consist of open ended questions. Possible questions could include:

1. What is working well for you in the course?
2. What could improve this course and make learning more effective?
3. Do you have any other suggestions for this current or future course?

(Stanford University, 2013)

NETIQUETTE

Netiquette, or Internet etiquette, is a type of guideline for posting and sending messages in the online classroom. Netiquette not only covers rules of behavior but also guidelines for ensuring interaction in the online environment. Shea (2011) outlined core rules of netiquette that every online student and instructor should follow:

- Remember the human (never forget there is really a person behind the keystrokes)
- Adhere to the same standards of behavior online that you follow in real life (in other words, be ethical)
- Know where you are in cyberspace (i.e., main discussion area, group forum)
- Respect each other's time and bandwidth (post appropriate messages)
- Make yourself look good online (check grammar and spelling)
- Share expert knowledge (help answer others' questions)
- Help keep tempers under control (don't respond to irate postings)
- Respect other people's privacy (do not read others private email)
- Don't abuse your power
- Be forgiving of other people's mistakes (you were once new to the online environment as well)

The core rules of netiquette were designed to help students who are new to the Internet to make friends instead of enemies. The instructor can post or link to these basic rules to help students understand the basic expectations of behavior online.

SPECIAL CONSIDERATIONS

Diversity and Americans with disabilities are global issues facing us daily and occur as well in the online environment. Since these issues are sensitive to many people, instructors should consider human equity issues seriously. Diversity consists of two dimensions, primary and secondary.

- Primary dimensions are those characteristics that everyone is born with and that are visible and easy to identify. They include age, gender, race, ethnicity, and other physical characteristics.
- Secondary dimensions are differences or characteristics that we acquire or change throughout our lives. These include work experience, income, marital status, religious beliefs, and education. These dimensions shape everyone we encounter in school, the workplace, and social settings (Center for Research on Education, Diversity and Excellence, 2012).

Government agencies, corporations, and educational institutions are now recognizing the necessity of valuing diversity to remain competitive and effective. As a facilitator, one needs to eliminate stereotypes and become more educated about different groups. This way, one is less likely to generalize. Suggestions for doing this might include:

- Becoming aware of the stereotypes you hold
- Determining the source of the stereotype and how it was formed
- Expanding your knowledge about other groups and cultures
- Expanding your experiences with other groups and cultures

Key Points of Americans with Disabilities Act

The Americans with Disabilities Home Page identifies security and testing issues in distance learning. They direct universities to make their distance learning classes accessible to qualified individuals with a disability, just as they are required to do for traditional courses. Specifically, Title 42 U.S.C. sec. 12132 states: "Subject to the provisions of this subchapter, no qualified individual with a disability shall, by reason of such disability, be excluded from participation in or be denied the benefits of the services, programs, or activities of a public entity, or be subjected to discrimination by any such entity." For nonpublic institutions, 42 U.S.C. sec. 12182 provides: "No individual shall be discriminated against on the basis of disability in the full and equal enjoyment of goods, services, privileges, advantages or accommodations of an entity" (American with Disabilities Home Page, 2013). These provisions protect and ensure Americans with disabilities equal access to online education and all information provided to the general public.

As universities and faculty expand their distance education offerings, they are finding that they must include the virtual equivalents of wheelchair ramps when building their online classrooms. They must accommodate, for instance, the student who is unable to see navigational graphics on a web page due to blindness and the student who cannot listen to a streaming audio lecture because of deafness. In fact, many students with disabilities find that most website technological extravaganzas are more of a burden than an aid.

For the most part, distance education students with disabilities can already get the equipment they need to make up for their impairments. Blind students can use software that reads online text aloud or produces a Braille message for the students to follow. Students who cannot move their arms easily can use adaptive equipment to manipulate the computer with other parts of their bodies. But some common features of the Internet make navigation difficult for people with certain disabilities. Text reading programs, for instance, are unable to recognize graphics. The problem is easily avoided if the programs can pick up and read aloud alternate texts that are placed behind the graphics, but not every website provides those texts. Sites with frames and tables (two commonly used features of web page design) tend to confuse those programs, which often read from left to right, ignoring the layout. An important issue is for universities to determine exactly what the law requires.

As an online facilitator, considerations for students with disabilities need to be taken on an individual basis. For example, if you know a student has a particular disability, you will need to take into account accommodations that may be necessary for the particular problem. It should be determined from the beginning exactly what the student's imitations are and what devices the student is using, if any; for example, TTY phones, screen readers, or voice recognition software. Allowing more time for test taking may be necessary, or allowance for leniency on spelling if you know a student is using voice recognition software. Check with your institution for policy regarding disabilities. If you are using audio files, for example, be sure to include a text version of the same information. If you are including web references, be sure to check their format (amount of graphics, use of frames) for accommodating screen readers. The bottom line is that everyone should have equal access to information.

FACULTY DEVELOPMENT

Effective training for online faculty is imperative in order for quality instruction to be delivered. This training may be 1 to 2 weeks in length and may be paid or unpaid (Bristol & Zerwekh, 2011). As it becomes more evident what quality online instruction looks like, it will be necessary to incorporate training on the competencies associated with quality instruction into a comprehensive faculty training program (Bigatel et al., 2011). Faculty preparation for teaching online measurably improves learning effectiveness and satisfaction (Moore, 1993). The ION's *Making the Virtual Classroom a Reality* and the *Master Online Teacher Certificate* programs provide online teachers the skills, understanding, and knowledge they need to be a successful online faculty. The ION's website (www.ion.uillinois.edu/resources/) provides institutions with tools and resources for developing their own programs for faculty training. Faculty training is becoming so critical that even itunes (itunes .apple.com/us/itunes-u/faculty-development-for-online/id421439101) and YouTube (www.youtube.com/watch?v=m3H7PbkndOk)) are posting faculty development snippets or brief training videos on developing an online course, fostering student interaction, distance learning and Web 2.0, and other topics.

THE SUCCESSFUL DISTANCE STUDENT

The student role in a distance course also changes significantly from a face-to-face classroom. Students must be more responsible for their own learning, be able to communicate through writing, and must possess certain characteristics that will ensure their ability to participate successfully in an online program. There is greater emphasis on identifying one's own learning needs and making plans to achieve learning objectives. In other words, online learning takes self-direction and discipline on the part of the distance student. The ION describes what the profile of a successful online student looks like (ION, 2013). Prior to becoming an online student, the individual must have some basic knowledge of information technology in order to participate in a distance course. Gilbert (2001) suggests that students start by asking:

- What is online learning and what is it like?
- Where can I find it and is it for me?
- What works in an online environment?
- What criteria make a good candidate for online learning?
- What are the advantages or disadvantages?
- How do I choose an online learning provider?
- How do I pick a curriculum?
- How can I get information about sources?
- What makes for a good distance program?
- Where do I start?
- How can I succeed?
- How can I manage the tools and equipment?

When designing distance learning academic programs, the basic characteristics of students should be considered. Their ages, interests, skill levels, academic preparedness, and career goals, for example, all should be considered. Much of the literature suggests that older students and adults are the primary participants in distance programs. In the United States, typical adult distance learning students are between the ages of 25 and 50. Many online learners are adult students with family and job responsibilities who require the flexibility of online learning in order to advance in their jobs or to earn their degrees. However, as more and more students become exposed to the online learning model, the traditional profile is changing.

In your online course, you may want to include reference links to resources and tips for your students to use to help them be more successful online learners. Many universities have information on their home page with tips for success in online courses. Clearly outlining expectations and characteristics of a successful online student can help students determine if the online environment will be a productive learning environment for them. Questionnaires for prospective students to use to assess whether they are good candidates for online learning can often be found on the university home page.

STUDENT EXPECTATIONS

Online students should expect that their instructor would provide the best learning environment possible. According to Faculty Focus (2011) students identified what instructors should demonstrate in the online classroom: respect, responsiveness, knowledge, good communication, approachability, organization, professionalism, engagement, and humor. With consistency in instructor delivery, students can anticipate and prepare their coursework based on expectations of how the instructor will run the course. When managing an online course, the faculty and the student play important roles. The faculty must plan for how the course will be managed based on student profiles, and the student must take responsibility for learning. A variety of characteristics including demographics, motivation, academic preparedness, and access to resources should be considered as important for an online learner.

In summary, course management covers a breadth of considerations, from student orientation, to discussion facilitation, to instructor feedback for students. It is interesting to note that each time an online course is taught, the instructor will note nuances or frequently asked questions that will help to prepare better for the next class. The time has come where the students, armed with experience in online learning, are starting to focus less on technology and management issues and more on course content.

REFERENCES

Americans with Disabilities Act (ADA). (2013). Retrieved January 28, 2013, from http://www.ada.gov/2010ADAstandards_index.htm

Bigatel, P., Ragan, L., Kennan, S., May, J., & Redmond, B. (2011). Identification of competencies for online teaching success. *Journal of Asynchronous Learning Networks, 16*(1), 59–77.

Bristol, T. J., & Zerwekh, J. (2011). *Essentials of e-learning for nurse educators.* Philadelphia, PA: A. Davis and Co.

Center for Research on Education, Diversity, and Excellence. (2012). Retrieved from http://www.cal.org/crede/

Chickering, A., & and Ehrman, S. (1996). Retrieved from http://www.tltgroup.org/programs/seven.html

Faculty Focus. (2011). Retrieved from http://www.facultyfocus.com/

Gilbert, S. (2001). *How to be a successful online student.* New York, NY: McGraw-Hill.

Going the Distance. (2013). Retrieved from http://www.onlinelearningsurvey.com/reports/goingthedistance.pdf

Illinois Online Network. (2013). Retrieved from http://www.ion.uillinois.edu/resources/tutorials/overview/elements.asp#The%20Facilitato%20r

Moore, M. (1993). Transactional distance theory. In D. Keegan (Ed.), *Theoretical Principles of Distance Education.* New York, NY: Routledge.

Palloff, R., & Pratt, K. (1999). Building learning communities in cyberspace: Effective strategies for the online classroom. San Francisco: Jossey-Bass Publishers.

Ryan, M., Hodson-Carlton, K., & Ali, N. (2005). A model for faculty teaching online: Confrmation of a dimensional matrix. *Journal of Nursing Education, 44*(8), 357–364.

Shea, V. (2011). Net etiquette. Retrieved January 28, 2013, from http://www.albion.com/netiquette/introduction.html

Smyth, E. (2011). Faculty focus. Retrieved from http://www.facultyfocus.com/articles/philosophy-of-teaching/what-students-want-characteristics-of-effective-teachers-from-the-students-perspective/

Stanford University. (2013). Retrieved from http://ctl.stanford.edu/teaching/midterm-student-feedback.html

Vitale, A. T. (2010). Faculty development and mentorship using selected online asynchronous teaching strategies. *Journal of Continuing Education in Nursing. 41*(12), 549–556. doi: 10.3928/00220124-20100802-02

TEN

Assessment and Evaluation of Online Learning

CAROL A. O'NEIL AND CHERYL A. FISHER

Assessing the learner involves gathering data to identify needs, ability, and progress. Assessment is student oriented and is used to place, promote, graduate, or retain students. Evaluation is a judgment made by comparing a behavior to a standard. Evaluation is the measurement of a behavior and the comparison of that behavior to a predetermined expectation.

ASSESSMENT, EVALUATION, AND PEDAGOGY

Pedagogical theory forms the framework for the design of a learning experience. The learning experience is a process that starts with the purpose of the course. The objectives are developed from the purpose, with a logical flow from the purpose to the objectives. The learning strategies logically flow from objectives and, as well, the evaluation appropriately flows from the objectives. For example, if an instructor uses behavioral theory to design a learning experience, one would expect to see learning objectives that focus on the targeted behavior

131

and strategies that include rewards and consequences. The objectives and strategies drive the evaluation activities. If the learning objective is to state five signs and symptoms of congestive heart failure, the evaluation should measure whether the learner can do so. To determine if the student has achieved this objective, the student may be asked to name the five signs and symptoms or answer a multiple-choice question related to the topic.

TRADITIONAL ASSESSMENT AND EVALUATION

A traditional evaluation design measures the attainment of learning objectives through exams, papers, and projects that the student submits to the instructor. The instructor uses criteria to grade the student's assignments and to categorize them into a grade of A, B, and so forth. The student demonstrates learning as stipulated in the objectives, and based on the degree of attainment of those objectives, a grade is assigned. This is called norm referenced assessment, because we make judgments about learning and a bellshaped curve is an expected outcome. This means that some students get grades of D or F, others get A grades, and the mean is about a B or C. The students are responsible for their learning and their grade. Another type of assessment is criterion referenced, which is based on learning for the purpose of meeting a standard. In this type of assessment, the instructor is responsible for helping all learners meet the standard. An example of a standard is validation, such as CPR validation.

In addition to the students, traditional evaluation includes gathering data about the course from an end-of-course survey that is completed by students. The administrator compiles the data and gives the results to the faculty to review. Data may be used to make changes in the course delivery before the course is offered again.

Traditional assessments may also include measuring the students' progress through a course or on the way to completing the course. Usually assessment techniques are process oriented and might take the form of a quiz. The purpose of assessment is to check the progress of students to identify those who may be struggling through the course.

CONSTRUCTIVISM AND ONLINE LEARNING

When constructivism is the guiding theory in learning, students construct new knowledge by actively engaging in learning strategies. Students reflect on the learned content and their reflections bring meaning to a larger social context or to solve real-world problems. Learning is process oriented, and when basic knowledge is used to construct new knowledge, the basic knowledge is reinforced. Traditional evaluation designs predominantly focus on measuring the students' achievement of objectives. Online learning evaluation should focus on the students' achievement of objectives and the new knowledge that was constructed during the learning process. While learners are constructing new knowledge, they need feedback. Feedback means that learners need comments from teachers that will motivate them to continue constructing knowledge or to continue moving in a constructive direction.

A traditional evaluation design does not accommodate the use of technology as a learning tool. Let us say that a student registers for an online course and shows up at the faculty's office the second week of the semester asking where the class will be held. Somehow, the student already has missed information and thus progress is hampered. By the second week of the semester, the student should have the computer skills needed to negotiate the online course, should have the needed resources (i.e., course entry information such as user name and password), and should know how to navigate through the course. If the student does not have these basic skills, the student will have to spend time learning navigational skills instead of course material. To get the student directly into the learning material, pre-course student assessments should be planned into the design of the learning experiences.

These assessments should provide data about the student's readiness to take a course online. Data gathered about student readiness should be summarized and a prescriptive plan developed that will guide the learner to resources needed to be successful online. The prescriptive plan is written and individualized for each student and includes activities and outcomes that focus on the skills that will ensure success online. Some examples include: knowing how to download files, navigating the web, receiving and sending email, sending attachments, and basic typing skills.

When developing learning material online, the learning material should be peer reviewed before it is released to learners. Peer review is a process in which a designated reviewer uses established criteria to review a course. Information gathered from the review is shared with the course developers so corrections can be made before students log on to the course. A peer review is crucial for newly developed courses, because there may be links that do not work, spelling and grammatical errors, or even exam dates in the syllabus that are not the same as the dates on a calendar. The purpose of a peer review is to enhance the quality of learning for the student. The reviewer has a "fresh set of eyes" that can detect errors so they can be corrected before the learners arrive. It is recommended that peers review or follow a course while it is offered to students.

Faculty should be recognized for their contributions and successes when they teach online. Faculty who teach online should request that content and technology experts "sit in" on their courses as guests to provide feedback. This feedback can be used for tenure and promotion, to promote recognition of scholarship of teaching and learning online, and to provide visibility for online courses, especially to faculty who do not teach online.

Technology influences on the course before it is offered, while it is being offered, and at the end of the course. Online learners need an orientation to the technology and learning platform before the course starts. Evaluating the effectiveness of the orientation is important for revising and refining. During the course, servers can crash and hard drives can go down. For example, during one semester, students were assigned to gather secondary data about a community. Data about the behavioral indicators of a community, such as smoking, obesity, prenatal care, and so forth, were located on a server that was managed by the state health department. About a week before starting content on the community assessment module, the information was pulled offline by the state health department. The faculty checked the links to this website before the course started, and therefore did not know that the link was not working when the students were given the assignment.

Evaluating the online course while it is live is essential. Early in the course, the faculty can ask students to email them with anything that looks like a course issue as soon as it becomes apparent. Give students permission to ask "dumb" questions like "Should the syllabus icon link to the syllabus?" Faculty needs information to quickly correct whatever glitches may arise. Aside from technical issues, there could be learner issues. Conflicts between students may develop or there could be hurt feelings because someone typed a comment that was read as negative. A quick response to technical and student issues while the course is running prevents further (and usually more chaotic) repercussions. At the end, the course needs to be evaluated by faculty, learners, and instructional designers using tools that focus on gathering data that are particular to online courses.

SUMMARY OF TRADITIONAL VS. ONLINE ASSESSMENT AND EVALUATION

In summary, evaluation of online learning differs from that of traditional classroom learning. Assessing the learner is an essential component in online learning. Learners' skills and abilities and responses to orientation need to be assessed, learners need feedback during the course while they are constructing new knowledge, and they need grades assigned at the end of the course. Therefore, traditional assessment and evaluation models need to be revised to accommodate learning online.

FOUNDATIONAL KNOWLEDGE OF ASSESSMENT AND EVALUATION

Smith and Ragan (2005) use the term "evaluation." They offer two purposes of evaluation: to assess individual student's performances and to provide information to revise course material. They call evaluation a way of "getting there": Did the student "get there" and how well did the instruction get the student there? They suggest that assessments be based on the learning objectives and called criterion referenced assessment items. Their purpose is to assess competence or to identify gaps in learning, but they do not compare or rank learners. That is the purpose of norm referenced tests. Smith and Ragan write that assessments are either criterion or norm referenced, thus alluding to two types of assessment: to identify gaps and to compare students' learning.

Smith and Ragan describe three types of assessments: entry skills assessments, pre-assessments, and post-assessments. The entry skills assessment focuses on skills needed to be successful in the online course, pre-assessments focus on ascertaining what the students already know, and post-assessments focus on attainment of learning objectives. They outline the characteristics of good assessment instruments as valid, reliable, and practical. A valid assessment answers the question: Does it measure what it claims it will measure? A reliable instrument is one that yields consistent outcomes over time. A practical assessment is cost effective. Smith and Ragan (1999) suggest two formats of assessment: performance assessment and paper-and-pencil tests.

These authors further describe evaluation as a means of providing information to revise course material and offer two types of evaluation: formative and summative. Formative evaluations provide information for the purpose of revising the instruction, and summative evaluations provide data about the continued use of the instruction.

NEW MODEL FOR ASSESSING AND EVALUATING ONLINE LEARNING

The authors of this book developed a model that incorporates the foundations of assessment and evaluation, guided constructivism, and online learning. The following questions were asked: Did the teaching methods and strategies used in this learning experience effectively impart information? Did the recipients learn the information? These questions are answered when assessing student learning and evaluating the course.

Assessment and evaluation are activities that are planned when the course is designed. The activities should be appropriate and congruous measures of the goals and objectives of the course. The activities provide data that can be used to make judgments about student learning and course effectiveness. Data can be gathered about the feasibility of student success online, the progress of the student through the course, student achievement of the course objectives at the end of the course, the effectiveness of the course design, the effectiveness of the course while it is taught, and the outcomes of the course. Student learning and course functioning are two aspects that need to be addressed separately. A model is suggested that will focus on student learning and course evaluations separately.

Assessment focuses on the student, and evaluation focuses on the course. Assessment and evaluation are built into the course design and are visible throughout the course from before the beginning of the course until after the course ends.

Assessment is defined as the identification of student needs and progress throughout the learning experience. The purpose of pre-course assessments is to identify the needs of the student so they can be remediated before the course begins. During the course, the focus is on the students' progress. The faculty monitors the students throughout the course and gives feedback about the process of constructing new knowledge. Assessing the learner at the end of the course is determined by graded activities. Grading criteria should be clearly specified in the syllabus.

Evaluation focuses on the course itself. Pre-course evaluation includes peer review of the course and an evaluation of the orientation program that is given to students before they enter the course. Formative evaluation is directed at how the course is operating, and summative evaluation is evaluation of the course after it is completed.

A new model called the Model for Assessing and Evaluating Learning Online, as seen in Figure 10.1, was developed based on Smith and Ragan (1999). The aspects of achievement are divided into three phases for student assessment and three phases of course evaluation.

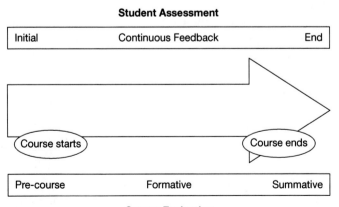

Student Assessment

| Initial | Continuous Feedback | End |

Course starts   Course ends

| Pre-course | Formative | Summative |

Course Evaluation

FIGURE 10.1   The model for assessing and evaluating learning online.

During each phase, evidence is gathered and analyzed. At each phase decisions are made based on the analyzed evidence. For example, at the end of the initial phase of student assessment, a prescriptive plan is developed that outlines knowledge and competencies that the student needs to master to continue in the course. During the continuous assessment, students are given feedback and motivation to help them determine their progress. The end student assessment is the measure of individual achievement. Evidence is gathered about the student's ability to meet objectives, and a decision to pass or fail is determined.

STUDENT INITIAL ASSESSMENT

Researchers have identified various types of initial student assessment techniques. Faculty and course developers can use these techniques to determine a range of student skills from comfort with technology to preferred learning styles. The following list includes some suggestions for faculty to use when conducting an initial student assessment prior to participating in an online course:

- Initial letter of assessment about the student as a learner
- Placement exams
- Students develop personal web pages
- Electronic meeting
- Computer skills exercise
- Pretests
- Scavenger hunt to assess navigation skills (develop a scavenger hunt list and posting of announcements; ask students to find the items and email the answers to the instructor)
- Learning style surveys
- Readiness surveys
- Continuous feedback

Continuous student feedback can be conducted at any time during the course. The purpose of continuous feedback is to determine if the student is learning from the course material presented. It is important for the faculty to know if the lectures and content of the course have been presented in a clear and logical format. Obtaining this information prior to the end of the course enables the instructor to make changes. Some of these techniques include:

- Journaling, writing marathons, diaries: These techniques assess attitude and satisfaction (affective objectives)
- Creating written logs about experiences and reflections
- Concept mapping: connective key concepts
- Giving mid-semester assessment
- Estimating student time ranges for each assignment plus interaction
- Giving feedback
- Having 3-minute "things I don't understand about" sessions
- Assigning a weekly new idea
- Debating
- Asking students to answer the question: What was the fuzziest point?
- Assigning reaction paper
- Assigning worksheets
- Giving nongraded quizzes
- Using simulations
- Assigning crossword puzzles
- Tracking attendance
- Allowing peer questions to other students
- Encouraging participation in discussion board
- Assigning homework
- Questioning
- Assigning case studies, which are detailed accounts of a client, family, group (e.g., pregnant teens), or community
- Completing a student assessment

At the end of a course, students are assessed in terms of meeting the course learning objectives. Multiple methods can be used and the following list identifies some methods:

- Quizzes
- Compositions, essays, and papers
- Projects (individual or group); project summaries, webpage presentations
- Analysis of newspaper article
- Examinations: Exams can be multiple choice and/or essay. They can be timed and proctored to ensure that students submit their own work. Students can take exams in schools of nursing, at outreach sites, at community colleges with faculty proctors, at local libraries, or at home with approved proctors. Exams can be proctored at

testing centers such as the Sylvan Learning Centers. Proctoring by video may also be an option.

- Portfolios (efolios): These are collections of student work in the course stored in a digital medium such as a flash drive. The work may include reflective essays, patient care plans, pamphlets developed for a health fair, pictures of a health project at an immunization fair, or an audiotape of a song about preventing teen pregnancy.
- Student presentations
- Peer evaluation
- Final interviews
- Rubrics

Rubrics are sets of standards that can be used to assign grades and give students feedback about their performance. Rubrics can use descriptions or commentaries on achievement, such as excellent, good, fair, or poor or they can be numerical. Many rubrics are online and can be found at the Rcampus Rubric Gallery (www.rcampus.com/rubricshellc.cfm?sms=publicrub&sid=35&).

PRE-COURSE EVALUATION

Pre-course evaluations help faculty determine if the course is ready for launching. Ideally, an external, objective reviewer should review the course for content and for instructional design. The peer reviewer should then continue to observe the course for interaction approximately 2 weeks into the course and again at midterm. The reviewer provides constructive feedback to the instructor, which can be used to make changes in the course. Pre-evaluation activities can include:

- Peer review of content
- Peer review of design

FORMATIVE EVALUATION

Formative evaluation throughout the course allows the faculty to determine if course delivery, structure, or instructional design needs revising. For example, students may ask for a discussion forum to list technology issues and ask for peer help. By providing students with the opportunity to ask questions during the course, issues can be resolved quickly and students can focus on their learning. Some suggestions for formative evaluation are:

- "Pulse Check": Ask students on a regular basis, maybe every 4 weeks or 3 times during the semester, to post or email their "pulse"— where they are and how they are doing in the course—and what improvements or changes they think should be made
- Discussion summaries every other week about course content and issues
- Mid-semester survey
- Verbal feedback to specific questions
- Summative Evaluation: The institution often requires summative evaluation. This evaluation provides feedback to the faculty to revise the course and to evaluate the faculty.

Examples include:

- Student evaluation of the course
- Student evaluation of faculty
- Faculty evaluation of the course

An overview of assessment strategies can be found in a Faculty Focus Special Report found at www.facultyfocus.com/wp-content/uploads/images/AssessingOnlineLearning-OC.pdf. The report includes 12 articles from Online Classroom and features such topics as mistakes to avoid, creating better multiple choice tests, and using self-check lists.

The Illinois Online Network offers topics on assessment and evaluation, such as homework, rubrics, and cheating. The resources can be found at www.ion.uillinois.edu/resources/tutorials/assessment/index.asp.

There are resources available for evaluating online courses. One is the Southern Regional Education Board (SREB) Checklist for Evaluating Online Courses. The criteria include content (14 subcriteria); instructional design (19 subcriteria); student assessment (7 subcriteria); technology (13 subcriteria); course evaluation and management (7 subcriteria).

Another resource for evaluating online courses is Quality Matters (www.qmprogram.org/files/QM_Standards_2011-2013.pdf). There are 8 standards: course overview and introduction, learning objectives, assessment and measurement, instructional material, learner interaction and engagement, course technology, learner support, and accessibility. There are 41 substandards.

In summary, a model has been developed that can be used to assess student learning and evaluate the learning environment. It incorporates the foundations of assessment and evaluation, guided constructivism, and online learning. Students should be assessed before the course starts to determine needs and learning style, during the course to determine progress, and at the end of the course as a final assessment of attaining goals. The course is peer evaluated before it is opened to students. Frequent evaluation of the course while it is being offered help to identify problems and issues that can be remedied. Evaluating the course at the end provides data to revise the course and data that can be used in developing new courses.

REFERENCES

Smith, P., & Ragan, T. (2005). *Instructional* design (3rd ed.). New York, NY: John Wiley & Sons, Inc.

Southern Regional Education Board.(2008). Checklist for evaluating online courses. Retrieved from http://publications.sreb.org/2006/06T06_Checklist_for_Evaluating-Online-Courses.pdf

ELEVEN

Theoretical Considerations for Professional Education

CHERYL A. FISHER AND WILLIAM A. SADERA

The availability of technology-supported continuing education (CE) for medical professionals began emerging in the early 1990s. Since that time, physicians, nurses, and other health care professionals have continued to seek available technology-supported CE because of the convenience, accessibility, and flexibility that it affords the users. Telecommunications and distance learning technologies are not new, but the increased capabilities and potential to reach a larger audience have transformed how we deliver education and training. More importantly, it has expanded our capacity to respond to the need to keep health professionals' knowledge and experiences current. With a long history of serving isolated and remote learners, distance learning has now emerged as an effective, mainstream delivery method of education and training that provides flexible learning opportunities in response to the needs of learners.

Historically, the results of research have been ignored and have not been applied to continuing education courses. Although the findings of empirical studies are essential to the quality of the distance learning experience, administrators and faculty are only just now starting to apply the results. This chapter provides an overview of current theoretical

143

approaches to online learning in CE. The purpose of this chapter is to review the current best practices and discuss the application of sound pedagogy, effective design, and the theoretical approaches that inform the design. Finally, this chapter will culminate in a proposed model for integration of theoretical approaches, best practices, and pedagogy that can be used to design future CE learning environments.

DISTANCE-BASED CE

With the rapid expansion of CE offerings online, it is becoming imperative that sound pedagogical design and the integration of emerging technologies be appropriately applied to the learning environment. With the realization that lifelong learning is more than attending conferences, the potential for greatly expanding effective continuing medical education (CME) through the use of technology has never been more encouraging. With consideration or guidance from learning theories, a well-designed learning environment should be well suited to meet the needs of active working professionals and adults who benefit from the convenience of technology-supported CE. Given the factors addressed through the guidance of learning theory, combined with the convenience and flexibility afforded through online education, offerings in this format will only continue to increase. Along with the increasing demand and growing consumer experience with distance learning modalities, expectations for quality instruction, successful educational outcomes, and satisfying learning experiences will also increase. These observations are validated by other researchers who found a significant increase in satisfaction, learning, and motivation between two physician groups (one using computer-based training and the other face-to-face training).

As technology advances and CE expands in the direction of distance-based courses, online CE providers need to research and continually assess learning within these environments. Educational activities for hospital staff do not easily match with the health care professional's personal and working life. Online learning could make it easier for health care personnel to attend courses, but the feasibility and effectiveness of using distance learning to meet educational goals in health care institutions requires further evaluation.

Mazzoleni, Maugeri, Rognoni, Cantoni, and Imbriani (2012) started an online educational program aimed at evaluating the impact of health care staff attendance as well as objective and subjective effectiveness. In a 15-month time frame, 5 e-learning courses were provided to 2,261 potential users at 14 hospitals, in parallel with traditional education. One thousand ninety-nine users from all the hospital have attended the courses (58% of nurses, 50% of therapists, 44% of technicians, 25% of physicians) for a total of 27,459 CME credits. Effectiveness in terms of knowledge gain was satisfactory and subjective evaluation was good (more than 95% satisfied users). E-learning is not always appropriate for all educational needs and is not a panacea, but the reported results point out that it may be an effective and economically convenient solution to support massive educational interventions, reaching results otherwise not attainable with traditional education (Mazzeleni et al., 2012).

In a review of 30 CE courses, quality of content was the characteristic most important to participants, and too little interaction was the largest source of dissatisfaction (Casebeer et al., 2004). More current research into networking and interactivity among practitioners is providing new information that has the potential to enhance the effectiveness of practice improvement. Insights from learning theories can provide a framework for understanding emergent learning resulting from interactions among individuals in trusted relationships such as online communities of practice. Failure to take advantage of practitioner interactivity may explain, in part, why some practice improvement study results show low rates of effectiveness. Examples of improvement models that explicitly use relationship building and facilitation techniques to enhance practitioner interactivity are now beginning to demonstrate effectiveness (Parboosingh, Reed, Caldwell, & Bernstein, 2011). Curricula to teach relationship building in communities of practice and facilitation skills to enhance learning in small group education sessions are just starting to be explored.

Other indications that interactivity and engagement may be key factors to successfully designing CME have been described by Reed, Schifferdecker, and Turco (2012). These authors found that students who wrote personal learning plans as a part of their CME experience were "very close" or "extremely close" to accomplishing their learning goals following the training. This demonstrates that distance-based

CE can be effective, but it is the design of these courses that needs to be carefully scrutinized to ensure a successful learning experience. These results corroborate previous research that has found "use of specific strategies to implement research-based recommendations seems to be necessary to ensure that practices change." The CE developers are responsible for responding to the needs of professionals to design, deliver, and evaluate new approaches to course design in order to determine the effectiveness of meeting the required outcomes.

As of 2012, a review of online CME instruction by Sklar (www.cmelist.com/instruction_Types_defined.htm, 2012) revealed that the most traditional format for CME delivery is still text based, followed by text and graphics, slide presentation or slides and audio, text and audio, guideline based, and others. This review indicates that over the past years, there continues to be an unsophisticated approach to CE design despite research findings. This trend, however, is that this is slowly beginning to change.

PEDAGOGY AND CONTINUING EDUCATION

Because the primary audience for CE comprises busy, working adult learners, institutions should ideally show consideration for these learners so that they have a choice in the organization and delivery of the learning program. During their careers, these professionals need a range of topics in CE to enhance their clinical skills and knowledge while providing care to patients. Specifically, the aim of most CE is to help improve practices and behaviors in order to provide the best quality care to patients and to maintain currency in practice. Nurses and physicians specifically require CE for acquiring new knowledge, skills, and attitudes that must be learned in order to keep pace with changes in practice. Traditional continuing professional education is taught through passive activities, such as lectures, face-to-face classes, and seminars. This kind of professional education usually requires the participants to be in the same place at the same time, which often does not coincide with the time demands of busy, working professionals. Schools have traditionally provided CE through media such as lectures, audio and video tapes, and printed monographs. Over the years, similar distance learning technologies and methods have been applied to the CME needs for rural and remote physicians. They have included audio teleconferencing, correspondence study, and compressed video-conferencing. But providers have not adapted instructional strategies to meet the capabilities of the technology or the learners. The continued emergence, growth, and capabilities of the Internet, the web, and webinar technologies have provided new opportunities for providing CE into the mainstream of health professionals.

THE ADULT LEARNER AND CE

Adults, compared to children and teens, have distinct needs and requirements as learners. It should be noted that adult learning is not a unique and specific process. Instead, generalizations about "the adult learner" imply that people over a certain age form a homogeneous group. However, differences in culture, cognitive style, life experiences, and gender may be far more important to learning than age (Shannon, 2003).

Adult learners are autonomous and self-directed (Knowles, 1970). They learn best when actively involved in the learning process and when instructors serve as facilitators. They should be allowed to assume responsibility for presentations and group leadership. Adult learners should be guided to develop their own knowledge rather than supplying them with facts. They have accumulated a foundation of life experiences and knowledge that may include work-related activities, family responsibilities, and previous education (Knowles, 1970). They need, then, to connect learning to this knowledge and experience base. To help these learners do so, instructors should draw out participants' experience and knowledge and must relate theories and concepts to the participants while recognizing the value of experience in learning. Additionally, instructors should treat these adults as equals in experience and knowledge and allow them to voice their opinions freely in class (Knowles, 1970). Because of these characteristics, adult learning programs should capitalize on the experience of the participants and should adapt to the age range of the participants. The course offerings should also provide as much choice as possible in the organization of the learning program in order to make the learning most relevant.

SOCIAL INTERACTION AND CE

Social interaction has long been thought to increase collaboration and, therefore, result in increased learning. One research study found that groups participating in social interaction were more satisfied and performed better on outcome measures (Jung, Choi, Lim, & Leem, 2002). In this study, the collaborative interaction group expressed the highest level of satisfaction with their learning experience, and the collaborative and social interaction groups participated more actively in posting their opinions than the academic interaction group. The conclusions of this study are in line with the aforementioned needs of the adult learner.

Interaction has less to do with personal interaction (e.g., building a community of learners) and more to do with providing a means of reinforcing various elements from the content of the training (Giguere, Formica, & Harding, 2004). This interaction has been recognized as one of the most important components of learning experiences both in conventional education (Vygotsky, 1978) and distance education (Moore, 1993). Research has shown that learning in groups improves students' achievement of learning objectives. Vygotsky (1978) believes that cognitive development and learning are dependent on social interaction. The major theme of his theoretical framework is that social interaction plays a fundamental role in the process of learning.

A second aspect of Vygotsky's theory is the idea that the potential for cognitive development is limited to a certain "time span," which he refers to as the zone of proximal development (ZPD). It is during this time that consciousness is raised and a range of skills can be developed with adult guidance or peer collaboration. Vygotsky's methods of analysis and conclusions about the development of human thought and language are still well regarded today and can be applied to the study of computer-mediated communication (Bacalarski, n.d.). Given the potential interactive nature of online learning environments and the needs of adult learners, the connections between these theories and this population are self-evident. This theory is discussed in more detail in Chapter 2.

CONSTRUCTIVISM

Constructivism is a theory of learning and an approach to education that emphasizes the ways that people create meaning through individual constructs. Constructs are the ways in which we interpret our realities to change our reality from chaos to order. Constructivism is a continual and sympathetic observation of students' interests and educational needs (Dewey & Archambault, 1964). As educators, this obligates us to continuously provide students with learning opportunities that support the exploration of ideas. In CE, this requires additional thoughtfulness since the learners possess such a rich background of experience and knowledge. Some examples of ways to incorporate constructivism into online CE include the incorporation of opportunities to give guided control to the learner. Some of the teaching models that can be utilized include cognitive apprenticeship, minimalist training, intentional learning environments, and case- or problem-based instruction. These models lend themselves well to medical content and can be utilized to make learning meaningful. Other elements (PSU, 2013) of this theory can be applied through design by:

- Allowing students to be responsible for their own learning
- Allowing students to determine what they need to learn
- Enabling students to manage their own learning activities
- Creating a nonthreatening setting for learning
- Making maximum use of existing knowledge
- Anchoring instruction in realistic settings
- Providing multiple ways to learn content
- Use of activities to promote higher-level thinking
- Encouraging creative and flexible problem solving
- Proving a mechanism for students to present their learning
- Using strategies that promote student responsibility

(Penn State University, 2013)

PEDAGOGICAL CONSIDERATIONS

Several key pedagogical considerations can be noted in the distance learning and CE literature based on the above theoretical approaches. Although distance education programs enhance access to CE for the health professional, increased access is often coupled with decreased quality in course design. According to Carriere and Harvey (2001), good course quality must take into consideration an understanding of the experiences of the providers. As a result of this need for understanding, a web-based survey aimed at CE providers was constructed to elicit a description of the providers, users, and the activities offered. This study revealed that participants had considerable interest in distance education development. Since distance CE features are now better known, this is a step toward the advancement and development of more and better distance programs as organizations share their experiences and models for programs.

Dolcourt, Zuckerman, and Warner (2006) noted competing time demands, irrelevant topics, and inconveniences such as parking and inclement weather as major factors for poor attendance at CE offerings in traditional formats. Improved accessibility, affordability of distance education, and time efficiency compared to the traditional conference-type programs are often cited as the primary reasons for offering distance-based CE. CE providers are well aware of professionals' busy schedules and are trying to accommodate their needs by offering ease of access and time efficiency. As consumers of educational products, busy health care providers make choices among competing alternatives for their time. By recognizing key decision factors, CE developers can potentially increase attendance and satisfaction by structuring style, content, and logistics to better accommodate the learners' perspectives.

IMPROVING QUALITY BASED ON EVIDENCE

Better programs would not be possible without consideration of practitioner experiences that suggest that interacting with peers and mentors in the workplace provides the best environment for learning, which, in turn, enhances professional practice and professional judgment (Parboosingh, 2011). This assertion is supported by research findings that reaffirm two important principles in adult learning. First, we learn most naturally when faced with meaningful problem-solving experiences; second, learning results in action when constructed by the individual. Without sound pedagogical principles and theoretical considerations for interaction and learner experiences, quality distance CE will not be possible (Parboosingh, 2011).

Although the trend is to put more and more CE online, it has only been recently that pedagogical considerations for design and delivery are starting to be noted (Fisher & Sadera, 2011). For example, in recent years CE developers were looking at interactive strategies to enhance learning using activities such as "blogging" or reflective journaling. A study by Bouldin, Homes, and Fortenberry (2006) found that although reflective journaling can be used as a learner-centered assessment tool to determine whether students are actually making sense of the content discussed in class, the students described this activity as "busy work." This demonstrates the need for interaction to be an integral part of the course design, not just an added activity. This notion was validated by a study in 2011 by Fisher and Sadera who found that if the mechanisms for interactivity are not integral (i.e., optional), then the learners are less likely to utilize them and therefore will not benefit.

Davis, O'Brien, and Freemantle (1999) reviewed randomized controlled trials on CE interventions and found personal interaction to be central to effective change in practice. Several studies reported that health care professionals seek confirmation and validation of current and new medical practices through their peers. Other studies have confirmed the importance of interaction in changing professional behavior. However, researchers have not established which elements of the interactive process enable learning. This is despite the preference shown among physician groups that many prefer lectures, although this may include interaction if it is built into the design of the class in a meaningful way to build knowledge.

Learning and practice cannot be separated when professionals work closely in specialty areas within the health care arena (Parboosingh, 2011). Interestingly, however, physicians report that such interactions with colleagues are an important source of learning, and educators and course designers have only recently considered using the power of communities to foster learning through practice (Parboosingh, 2011). Membership within a learning community, however, has its responsibilities, because expectations and pressures from peers and mentors in a community of practice influence standards for learning and practice. The significance of this finding tells us that continuing professional development providers should focus on meeting the learning needs of multidisciplinary communities of practice rather than individual learners. This research has implications for design considerations of CE courses.

More acceptable and effective methods for professional continuing education should be required to promote health care team member collaboration. It is has been argued that this collaboration would then encourage health care workers to interact with peers and mentors in order to frame issues, brainstorm, validate and share information, make decisions, and create management protocols, all of which contribute to learning in practice (Parboosingh, 2011). Physicians, however, were quick to note that if the CE was not directly related to their practice, then it would be a waste of their time.

CE AND QUALITY EDUCATION

As distance-based CE has grown steadily over the past several years, the quality has received limited attention in the medical literature, and few have attempted to establish or describe quality standards (Olson & Shershneva, 2004). Standards can be used to synthesize practical knowledge, best practices, and research findings. They vary in their perspectives on quality, fall short of being comprehensive, and convey many elements that apply to distance CE. The conclusions are that published standards in the distance education literature can provide valuable guidance to distance CE providers, and additional research questioning what works in CE and why is clearly needed. The standards should be seen as instruments to achieve a higher goal while remaining cognizant of what is trying to be achieved.

A framework for implementing technology-enabled knowledge translation into the health care culture was described by Ho et al. (2004). They claim that cultivation and acceptance in the domains of perceiving types of knowledge and ways in which clinicians acquire and apply knowledge in practice are required. Ho et al. (2004) argue that in order for knowledge transfer to take place, the following issues need to be met: understanding the conceptual and contextual frameworks of information and communication technologies as applied to health care systems; comprehending essential issues in implementation of information and communication technologies as well as strategies to take advantage of emerging opportunities; and finally, establishing a common and widely acceptable evaluation framework. The successful transfer of knowledge from a technology-supported learning environment to practice, according to these authors, depends on: a vision about the goals to be achieved; identification of cultural and political issues, and human and financial resources; as well as addressing legal, ethical, and technological limitations. This framework takes into account the complex considerations of CE design coupled with technology and the ultimate purpose for delivery being that of change in practice.

New developments in technology allow today's CE providers to more effectively meet the criteria necessary for effective CE. These factors include convenience, relevance, individualization, self-assessment, independent learning, and a systematic approach to learning. A case study conducted at the International Virtual Medical Schools in the United Kingdom (Harden, 2005) demonstrated how rapid growth of distance learning can alter undergraduate education and can have the potential to alter the nature of CE. Key components include a bank of reusable learning objects, a virtual practice with virtual patients, a learning outcomes framework, and self-assessment instruments. Learning is facilitated by a curriculum map, guided learning resources, "ask the experts" opportunities, and collaboration or peer-to-peer learning. Researchers (Harden 2011) also found that distance learning provided a bridge between the cutting edge of education and training and outdated procedures embedded in institutions and professional organizations. It is often these organizations that can be credited for keeping health care professionals up to date with current practice issues.

If health care professionals are not kept up to date with current practice, the design and subsequently the quality of CE course offerings are only going to deteriorate. Without the keen attention and deliberate actions for incorporating research findings into new course design, health care practitioners will ultimately not be achieving their goal of knowledge enhancement for the ultimate purpose of providing current, up-to-date patient care.

STRATEGIES FOR IMPROVING CE

Problem-solving strategies illustrate the contribution of theory to practice. The ability to frame and solve problems is central to the health care professional's level of competence. It is known that the ability to solve problems is tightly tied to one's knowledge in that area; therefore, problem-solving ability varies markedly from case to case and from context to context. These findings have led to new understandings and revised theories about promoting the learning of problem solving. We now know that learners require a wide variety and number of opportunities along with exemplars in learning how to solve problems so that they have many different strategies and approaches in their arsenal. The iterative relationship between theory and practice provides a powerful tool for improvement in the field.

Additional principles that should be applied to CE design should include Chickering and Gamson's (1987) and Chickering and Ehrman's (1996) seminal work. These principles should be incorporated into the pedagogical design utilizing opportunities for active learning strategies, feedback, time on task, and efficiency of delivery utilizing technology, collaboration with peers, interaction with faculty, setting high course expectations, and showing respect for diversity. The model shown in Figure 11.1 depicts an approach for incorporating the multifaceted considerations necessary when designing quality CE. This model considers principles for adult learning, layered with considerations for the experiential learner, specifically in health care, in addition to the opportunity for social interaction, since this is known to support learning. This interaction could be technology supported, coupled with best practices for teaching with technology. Evaluation should also be built into the course design, because it is well documented that this area is also often overlooked in CE relative to practice change.

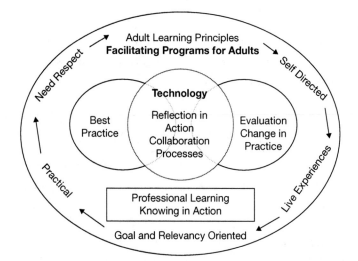

FIGURE 11.1 A model for CE design utilizing layered theory, best practices, and evaluation.

SUMMARY

The purpose of this chapter was to identify a multifaceted pedagogical approach for distance-based CE from a theoretical perspective as evidenced by the distance learning and the CE literature. This chapter also addressed current empirical studies on distance-based CE, which are also now starting to look at pedagogical design considerations by incorporating opportunities for interaction and principles. Several theoretical components can be applied in order to explain and support future design of technology supported courses; however, this design must be cost efficient and must demonstrate positive outcomes. With the improvement in technology, computer and web-based education have set the stage for dynamic, information-rich learning opportunities.

The importance of technology to health care professional development is growing rapidly and is echoed throughout the literature. Access to distance CE must be immediate, relevant, credible, easy to use, cost efficient, and effective. A sense of high utility demands content that is focused and well indexed in order to meet the health care professional's needs. The roles of the CE provider must be reshaped to include helping health care professionals seek and construct the kind of knowledge they need to improve patient care.

Distance-based CE currently lacks a theoretical underpinning, does not consider best practices for teaching, and does not utilize technology to enhance the quality of course offerings. Current research should apply what is known from the field of educational research coupled with what is known about the health professional as learner in an attempt to deliver quality learning opportunities with better outcomes for practicing health care providers.

REFERENCES

Bacalarski, C. (n.d.). Vygotsky's developmental theories and the adulthood of computer mediated communication: A comparison and an illumination. Retrieved from http://psych.hanover.edu/vygotsky/bacalar.html

Bouldin, A., Holmes, E., & Fortenberry, M. (2006). Blogging about course concepts: Using technology for reflective journaling in a communications course. *American Journal of Pharmaceutical Education, 70*(4), 84.

Carriere, M., & Harvey, D. (2001). Current state of distance continuing medical education in North America. *Journal of Continuing Education in the Health Professions, 21,* 150–157.

Casebeer, L., Kristofco, R., Strasser, S., Reilly, M., Krishnamoorthy, P., Rabin, A., Zheng, S., Karp, S., & Myers, L. (2004). Standardizing evaluation of online continuing medical education: Physician knowledge, attitudes, and reflection on practice. *Journal of Continuing Education in the Health Professions, 24,* 68–75.

Chickering, A., & Ehrmann, S. (1996, October). Implementing the Seven Principles: Technology as lever. *AAHE Bulletin,* 3–6.

Chickering, A., & Gamson, Z. (1987, June). Seven principles for good practice in undergraduate education. *AAHE Bulletin.*

Dewey, J., & Archambault, R. (1964). *John Dewey on education: Selected writings.* New York, NY: Modern Library.

Dolcourt, J., Zuckerman, G., & Warner, K. (2006). Learners' decisions for attending pediatric grand rounds: A qualitative and quantitative study. *BMC Medical Education, 6*(26), 1–8.

Fisher, C., & Sadera, W. (2011). Comparing student learning and satisfaction between learning environments in continuing medical education. *International Journal of Instructional Technology and Distance Learning, 8*(5), 29–42

Giguere, P., Formica, S., & Harding, W. (2004). Large-scale interaction strategies for web-based professional development. *American Journal of Distance Education, 18*(4), 207–223.

Ho, K., Block, R., Gondocz, T., Laprise, P., Ryan, D., Thivierge, R., & Wenghofer, E.(2004). Technology-enabled knowledge translation: Frameworks to promote research and practice. *Journal of Continuing Education in the Health Professions, 24*(2), 90–99.

Jung, I., Choi, C., Lim C., & Leem, J. (2002). Effects of different types of interaction on learning achievement, satisfaction, and participation in web-based instruction. *Innovations in Education and Teaching International, 39*(2), 153–162.

Knowles, M. (1970). *The modern practice of adult education: Andragogy versus pedagogy.* New York, NY: The Association Press.

Mazzoleni, M., Maugeri, C., Rognoni, C., Cantoni A., & Imbriani, M. (2012). Is it worth investing in online continuous education for healthcare staff? *Studies in Health Technology Information, 180,* 939–943.

Olson, C., & Shershneva, M. (2004). Setting quality standards for web-based continuing medical education. *Journal of Continuing Education in the Health Professions, 24,* 100–111.

Parboosingh, J. (2002). Physician communities of practice: Where learning and practice are inseparable. *Journal of Continuing Education in the Health Professions, 22,* 230–236.

Parboosingh, J., Reed, V., Caldwell, J., & Bernstein, H. (2011). Enhancing practice improvement by facilitating practitioner interactivity: New roles for providers of continuing medical education. *Journal of Continuing Education in the Health Professions, 31*(2): 122–127.

Pennsylvania State University. (2013). Retrieved from http://www.ed.psu.edu/educ/in-sys

Reed, V., Schifferdecker, K. E., Turco, M. G. (2012). Motivating learning and assessing outcomes in continuing medical education using a personal learning plan. *Journal of Continuing Education in the Health Professions, 32*(4): 287–294.

Shannon S. (2003). Adult learning and CME. *The Lancet, 361*(9353), 266–266s.

Sklar, B. (2013). Online CME: An update. Retrieved January 2013, from http://www.cmelist.com/mastersthesis

Vygotsky, L. (1978). *Mind in Society: The development of higher psychological processes.* Cambridge, MA: Harvard University Press.

TWELVE

Practical Considerations for Nursing Professional Development Education

SUSAN BINDON

Nurses and clinical staff work in hospitals and other patient care settings that, by nature, require seemingly endless amounts of education. Newly hired staff are oriented to the organization, the department, and their specific role. Clinicians must stay abreast of the latest evidence and apply it to their practice. They need to be informed of regulatory changes, policy and procedure revisions, and equipment updates. They seek education or training on nonclinical aspects of their role, such as communication or leadership skills. Clinicians are also obligated to maintain competence with relevant technical skills, and often require education and practice to do so. Patients and their families expect competence and a nearly error-free environment in which to receive care. In many respects, learning continues and is part of daily life for clinicians. Hospital-based education quite literally picks up where academic or professional education leaves off and continues throughout one's career. Lifelong learning is a key component of safe, competent nursing practice. This chapter explores the incorporation of online learning in the staff development setting, how it impacts both educators and learners, and the outcomes that can be realized by doing so. Aspects of each of these elements make the use of online learning in the hospital setting a unique challenge.

The American Nurses Association (ANA) position paper on professional role competence (ANA, 2008) has stated that nurses and employers share responsibility for creating an environment conducive to competent practice. They further extend accountability to include the profession, professional organizations, credentialing and certification entities, regulatory agencies, and other key stakeholders. Nursing professional development (NPD) specialists play a key part in this arena, and are largely responsible for initial and ongoing education of clinical staff. These nurse educators use knowledge and skills in education theory, design, career development, leadership, and program management to support and facilitate lifelong professional development (National Nursing Staff Development Organization, 2010). The varied responsibilities and scope of practice require NPD specialists (sometimes referred to as staff development specialists) to work creatively, efficiently, and at a high level of competence in overlapping professional contexts—clinical practice and education. NPD educators have expertise in applying the education process to address learning needs and to facilitate learning. The education process closely resembles the six-step nursing process, and helps to organize one's thinking. First, NPD educators *assess* learning needs and identify baseline knowledge and skill levels. Needs assessments are commonly done via survey, observation, interview, pre-test, or learner self-assessment data. Educators then *validate* their assessment with stakeholders to *identify outcomes* that are realistic and attainable. At this stage, *planning* begins. Educators write learner-centered objectives and design content. They select teaching and evaluation strategies that support the objectives and desired outcomes. NPD educators then *implement* the education plan, and finally *evaluate* learners' achievement of objectives and the effectiveness of the overall plan. Lesson plans are useful in creating clear, succinct overview of objectives, content, teaching strategies, learning and evaluation activities, time frames, and necessary resources. Lesson plans also help to ensure consistency among presenters, serve to document NPD responses to learning needs, and provide a template for design of future versions of the class or course.

To briefly illustrate this process and how it might be used, consider the following scenario. Based on latest evidence and standards of care, an organization decides to implement a new patient identification process. The process includes the use of bar codes on patient wrist bands, medications, and records. NPD is asked to educate staff about the new process in time for go-live, just 2 months away. Using their needs assessment skills, educators might determine that all clinical staff (850 learners) require education. Content will focus on the need for the new bar codes, the intended outcome of the bar code technology, current patient identification policy, staff's responsibility when identifying patients, the use of the scanner, and resources for troubleshooting. The educators share this assessment with key stakeholders who agree to the scope, objectives, and target outcomes. Next, the educators decide to use a blended learning approach to this project. First, they design an online module including rationale for the change, the current policy, a video demonstrating use of the scanner, links to external resources and evidence on patient safety, and a short self-assessment or quiz. They pilot the module with representative learners, and determine that the learning level is appropriate for all. Educators also schedule multiple drop-in sessions over the upcoming weeks to demonstrate the use of the scanner and allow learners to practice. The module is assigned to all clinical staff by job title and code, communication is extended to learners regarding access and availability, and the module is opened. Course completion is tracked via the organization's learning management system (LMS) and reports are provided to stakeholders. Educators also plan to provide support on the units for 1 week after go-live to answer questions and ensure that learning has occurred. They then evaluate the efficiency and effectiveness of the plan using module completion data, unit observations, and incident report data on patient identification for the next quarter. In this scenario the use of a blended format and online learning module allowed NPD educators to reach a wide audience in a relatively short time period.

In addition to their role as educators, NPD specialists act as consultants for unit-based or system-wide projects, are recognized leaders within an organization, and act as catalysts for the translation of evidence into practice. They are often subject matter experts (SME) on a wide range of clinical, technological, and regulatory topics. In some cases, NPD specialists act as facilitators of the education process rather than the actual providers of specific information. This supports the notion that the clinical workplace requires NPD educators to be learning experts, not simply content experts (Billings & Halstead,

2005). In short, the role of NPD specialists is broad and is constantly evolving to meet the demands of the organization and the learners to whom they are accountable. In recent years, the role has grown to include the design, use, and evaluation of online learning in staff development. Shanley (2004) states the staff educator's role includes facilitating staff adoption of technology. Greater emphasis on the use of technology to facilitate learning, such as simulation, distance and web-based learning, was identified as an emerging trend for NPD educators in the 2010 NPD Scope and Standards of Practice (National Nursing Staff Development Organization, 2010). Use of newer educational methodologies, including computerized instruction, is recognized as an essential competency for NPD educators (Brunt, 2007).

LEARNERS

In contrast to an academic setting where students in a particular class have relatively similar goals and ability levels, a special challenge for NPD specialists is the variety of learners for which they may be responsible. Though often discussed, there is not a definitive "right size" span of control or ratio of learners to educators in NPD. Depending on the topic, identified learners can include professionals (nurses, physicians, therapists), unlicensed workers (technicians, support staff, environmental services), nonclinical staff (security, transportation, admitting), and students from many disciplines. Inherent among these learners is a wide range of learning styles, ages, cultural backgrounds, literacy levels, languages, and other learning preferences and abilities. Added to this is the challenge of reaching learners in a 24/7 environment where they potentially work irregular schedules and shifts. There is precious little time for clinical staff in particular to be away from patient care responsibilities to attend classes or take advantage of optional educational opportunities.

Learners in a clinical setting are, by and large, adult employees or volunteers. They are not necessarily students who pay tuition and expect instructors to cover material and assign grades. Employees are motivated quite differently than students. Internal motivators may include reaching personal goals such as becoming certified in a nursing specialty; external motivators may include increased salary or expanded opportunities. In some instances, employees engage in learning following a mandate from supervisors or the organization itself, and are largely motivated by a need to be "signed off." Determining the best way to engage busy, diverse, often stressed adults to complete mandatory training or elective courses presents a significant challenge for NPD specialists. Online learning approaches can help by offering convenient, flexible, and efficient options to NPD instructors' repertoire of teaching strategies.

ENVIRONMENT/SETTING

Education in hospital and academic settings differs in several ways. NPD educators are usually outstanding clinicians in a particular specialty who have an interest in education and may be certified as NPD educators. Some have advanced degrees with an education focus; others have no formal background in education. They are typically responsible for addressing staff learning needs across large areas. For instance, one educator may cover several nursing units within a service line (surgical, rehabilitation, perioperative), rather than a specific number of courses or credits within a defined program. NPD educators draft annual education schedules, but in contrast to academia, hospital-based education has no firm academic calendar. Rather, timelines are developed and changed as needs arise throughout the year. Within this framework, NPD educators must be ready to adjust and reprioritize at any time to address issues of patient safety, risk management, and other unexpected events requiring education. Usually unforeseen, it is nearly impossible to plan in advance for this type of just-in-time (JIT) training. It is difficult to develop and deliver a quality product given a short turnaround time. Learners have an equally hard time absorbing information when bombarded from several angles simultaneously. Wright (1998) suggests the one competency every nurse needs in order to survive in such a pressured environment is the ability to "learn on the fly." Finding needed resources and quickly learning the essentials when faced with the new or unfamiliar is the hallmark of this type of learning.

Depending on the size of the organization, education departments range from one generalist to dozens of highly specialized instructors. How departments are organized (centralized or decentralized) and whether education is viewed as a value added investment depend on the organization's leadership philosophy. These elements are mentioned as they can influence NPD teaching and communication strategies, access to resources, and ability to effect change such as implementation of online learning.

LEARNING THEORY

NPD practice is built on the principles of adult learning (National Nursing Staff Development Organization, 2010). Coupled with constructivist learning theory, adult learning principles also anchor the approach to online teaching for nurses and other clinical staff. Central concepts of constructivist theory include interaction, collaborations, autonomy, reflection, and experiential learning. Nurses build on the knowledge and experience they already have to build or construct new meaning. NPD educators need to consider how nurses learn, and be sure that online materials and exercises are meaningful, relevant, and practical. Content must be in the right "language" and at the right level for connections to be made. Learners must actively engage in the education process to build meaning and understanding that they can readily apply to real-world situations. In terms of course design and delivery, nurses expect clear directions, flexibility, self-pacing, intuitive navigation, logical progression, and easy access to resources as needed. Practical information, opportunities for self-checking, and feedback and rationale for assessments enhance learning and learner satisfaction.

INCORPORATION OF ONLINE LEARNING STRATEGIES IN NPD

Traditionally, NPD educators relied heavily on face-to-face classroom teaching for orientation and other content-dense courses. Classes vary in length from an hour to an all-day workshop or even to a multiple-session program. Shorter unit-based inservices can be useful for updating staff on new equipment, policies, or practices These teaching methods have been popular in staff development for decades, but are quickly losing favor and practicality as the clinical environment becomes busier and more complex than ever before (Haggard, 2011). Inservice attendance has declined significantly as staffing models become leaner, and the opportunity to carve out even 15 to 30 minutes of time away from patient care needs becomes more difficult (Chapman, 2006). Attendees are interrupted with questions, alarms, and calls, leading to a chaotic learning environment. Other common methods of education delivery in NPD include posters, self-learning packets, mobile learning carts, walking rounds, drop-in or open training sessions, proctored computer or skills labs, simulation, one-on-one precepted learning, pre- and posttests, surveys, demonstrations, journal clubs, and grand round presentations. Online learning and blended learning formats have gained acceptance as viable strategies in recent years, providing much needed creative alternatives to the traditional approaches. Choice of teaching strategy depends on subject matter, objectives, audience, time, resources, educator skill, and learners' preferred styles. Each of these methods has pros and cons.

Online learning strategies in NPD have been shown to increase efficiency, improve compliance, and maintain teaching effectiveness in clinical use (Chapman, 2006). Online learning strategies, employed in the right situations, allow NPD specialists to reach their audience quickly and conveniently. Puetz (1991) envisioned this impact over 20 years ago, claiming that using technology in staff development would be essential for productivity, efficiency, and cost effectiveness. NPD educators tackle topics ranging from unit-specific equipment changes to yearly competency assessment for clinical staff to The Joint Commission updates for all hospital employees. Each of these is unique and requires NPD educators to assess and validate needs, plan content and strategies, provide education, and evaluate the effectiveness of the program and the process itself. This is not a simple task. It takes time, money, and skills; resources that are already strained in a dynamic, unpredictable environment.

The Cleveland Clinic Foundation (CCF) NPD department and its partners developed an online curriculum and integrated LMS in 2003to assist with educating a massive number of employees on patient confidentiality regulations (Dumpe, Kanyok, & Hill, 2007). The LMS helped to manage the "three Rs" of system-wide education efforts—registration, routing, and reporting. Registration refers to assigning the right people to the right course or learning module, and is usually done via job title or job code. Determining who the "right" people are is a decision made jointly by educators and stake-holders at the outset of a project. Decisions are based on need, relevance, and appropriateness of the material. All staff, for example, may need customer service training, whereas only nurses, providers, and pharmacists may need drug interaction modules. Routing refers to access and decisions about how, when, and where courses will be open and available to learners. Reporting is the all-important process of tracking attendance, performance, and completion rates of learners from specific roles or units. These data are then used for course management as well as employee performance appraisals and regulatory recordkeeping. Use of the LMS and online curriculum allowed the CCF team to get the needed information to 18,000 employees in 2 months. A follow-up survey showed that over 75% of the users were satisfied with the experience, and more than 65% actually preferred the online strategy to classroom training.

TECHNOLOGY AND COMPETENCY ASSESSMENT

This successful launch led to the development of a sophisticated online approach to nursing competency assessment and validation. Maintaining nurse competency is a monumental, ongoing undertaking, particularly as technology influences practice at breakneck speed. Countless hours of educator and staff time are involved, increasing the use of overtime funds and driving up the costs. Competency validation in the past has been an extremely labor- and paper-intensive endeavor, often taking place in the form of multiple day long "fairs" involving learning stations, demonstrations, and manual signing of individual checklists. Despite the education challenges faced by health care organizations, the use of online technology to demonstrate competency for nurses in the acute care environment has only recently been explored (Gerkin, Taylor, & Weatherby, 2009). CCF painstakingly redesigned 24 annual competencies for online validation, adding interactive elements, quizzes, and other learner-centered activities. Modules were designed at different "levels" of assessment for specific roles. For example, restraint documentation responsibilities differ from registered nurse to nursing assistant, and learning materials must reflect that difference. As a result of the online approach, the competency assessment process was standardized and streamlined. A built-in user survey showed that 87% of licensed and unlicensed users were satisfied with the process, 92% felt that it was user friendly, and 87% were able to complete their requirements on their home unit, saving time and money and minimizing interruption to work flow (Dumpe, Kanyok, & Hill, 2007).

Another example demonstrating the usefulness of online education in NPD involves nurse preceptor preparation. Preceptors guide new nurses through orientation. They act as role models, teachers, and advocates. Nurse preceptors need education and support in this role, which is in addition to their patient care responsibilities. Finding adequate and convenient time to educate preceptors without disrupting patient care is a challenge for NPD educators. Phillips (2006) suggests that online preceptor education programs can assist preceptors to learn and adopt the role in a timely manner. Convenience and access are the main attractions of online learning for preceptors, and some suggest that the outcomes of an effective preceptor program, namely job satisfaction, retention, and recognition, can be met using online learning strategies.

OTHER USES OF TECHNOLOGY IN PROFESSIONAL DEVELOPMENT

Perhaps the activity that consumes the most NPD educator time is new employee orientation. Depending on the size of the organization, orientation takes place monthly or bi-monthly, and can range from 1 day to 2 full weeks of face-to-face classroom or blended teaching strategies. Incorporating online learning strategies shortens the length of hospital orientation time significantly. Many organization now use a blended approach, providing new employees with online information about the hospital mission and vision, benefits, review materials and tests, corporate compliance training, human resources policy links, and other general information for their review prior to starting a new job. NPD educators can also provide resources to help newly hired nurses prepare for a standard pre-hire medication calculation test. In such one instance, test scores improved dramatically (Payne, 2012). Onsite classroom time is then minimized, and time can be used instead to meet team members and supervisors, clarify questions, and review key points.

In an effort to gain efficiency and save money, e-classrooms are allowing educators to deliver a consistent, quality program built on information specific to the organization. Use of an e-classroom modality, in which learners collaborate and interact online both synchronously and independently, is driven by the need for more and more classroom time to cover material deemed as mandatory or critical for new employees. Online learning provides a way for educators to cover more material without adding additional time or costs. Depending on hospital policy, some learning can take place before employees report for orientation or outside of the hospital, thereby decreasing the need for class time. Classroom interaction is used to clarify information and address questions learners may have. Using online resources for orientation provides anytime access and allows for quick updating and revision of materials as changes occur. Printing costs are decreased and training materials are easier to manage. For example, NPD can provide new employees with a "highlights folder" instead of a full hard-cover binder of printed material (Payne, 2012). While the online approach to orientation took significant instructor time to design, build, test, upload, and manage, it eventually saved a great deal of time for both users and educators.

There are many opportunities to incorporate online learning in NPD besides new employee orientation. Continuing education (CE) is a key component of nursing practice and as such, often falls under the auspices of NPD. NPD educators are constantly challenged to create and provide creative, stimulating, up-to-date, cost-effective CE programs. Examples of CE include specialty courses such as chemotherapy certification preparation or advanced critical care courses, both of which are content rich and well suited for reconceptualization to online formats. These courses are offered repeatedly as the need arises or on an annual basis. Online links, resources, case studies, and practice questions can augment straightforward content, and discussion areas provide a way for learners to interact with instructors and each other. Thomas Jefferson University Hospital changed its traditional 2-day nursing classroom dysrhythmia course to an e-learning experience (Elkind, Wus, & Parra, 2008). NPD educators were one of the driving forces for the transformation of the course, the reinforcement of learning, and the acceptance of technology-based learning for future endeavors.

There are other examples of how online learning is changing the practice of NPD. Annual "mandatory" training in fire safety, infection control, and corporate compliance can be transferred with relative ease to an online format due to the factual and standard nature of the content. All employees, volunteers, and students must complete the modules annually in keeping with regulatory standards. Placing "mandatories" online and using a learning management system for assigning, tracking, and reporting employee compliance results in time and cost savings and ensures that all staff get the same information. Consideration must be made for follow up and resource identification in the event of questions. Support for nonreaders must also be addressed, such as planning for a minimal number of face-to-face classes on all shifts and weekends, or making audio-assisted versions of the learning module available. Accommodations must also be made for participants with disabilities. Specifics related to accommodating online learners are discussed in Chapter 9: Course Management Methods.

Other skill-based training is being converted to blended offerings as well. For example, the American Heart Association offers cardiopulmonary resuscitation (CPR) and advanced cardiac life support (ACLS) renewal training using a blended learning approach via Online AHA® (American Heart Association, 2013). Learners register for and complete didactic content online, then are required to pass an instructor-facilitated skills session before completing the course and receiving a course completion card. Again, instructor time is drastically reduced from 4 hours per class to 1 hour per skills validation session, and learners can access and interact with the material at their convenience. Depending on setting and hospital policy, CPR and ACLS certifications are annual or bi-annual events, necessitating massive amounts of time, space, materials, and instruction when using a traditional face-to-face format.

Online formats are also useful for sharing best practices, policies and procedures, blogs, and wikis. They are extremely helpful when working with students. Students must be welcomed and oriented to the clinical site and its electronic documentation system before starting their learning experience. They also have practical needs such as badging, parking, and security information. Large teaching hospitals can feasibly host over a thousand students per year, and the use of online resources can dramatically reduce orientation time and instructor demand.

Online learning has usefulness for NPD educators outside of the hospital. Nursing staff working in community settings also require education. It is impractical to arrange inservices and track attendance for staff who work across large geographic areas, require travel time, and manage sometimes unpredictable patient case loads. Online formats can allow nurses and other clinicians to access and participate in webinars and other learning events without travel time and cost. This is particularly useful in rural areas or settings that do not necessarily have access to universities, experts, and other cutting-edge resources. One home care agency, challenged with a way to streamline required yearly pain, end of life, and infection prevention education, chose to use an online approach. Flexibility, alignment with adult learning principles, and appeal to its mobile learners were key considerations for this decision. Staff compliance and course completion rates increased from an estimated 40% or 50% to 98% when the sessions were converted to online offerings. Data also showed a related improvement in satisfaction with staff education, up to 91% (Elliott & Dillon, 2012). Based on the success of online annual training, the agency moved to incorporate online competency education, orientation modules, and CE courses. The importance of computer skills, access, quality design, and thoughtful communication were recognized and highlighted, as was the need to provide one-to-one or small group training to nonreaders or those with limited computer abilities.

With all of its potential uses, online learning is not an automatic answer for all classes. NPD educators must still be mindful to appropriately align content and teaching strategies. Since some online learning is static and one way, sensitive issues like intimate partner violence or removing life support may not be best suited for an all-online format, particularly if presented in self-learning modules or if learners and instructor are present asynchronously (Klingbeil, Johnson, Totka, & Doyle, 2009). If sensitive topics are going to be offered online, they should be presented with an opportunity for discussion.

DECISION POINTS FOR USE OF ONLINE LEARNING STRATEGIES IN NPD

Stakeholders must quickly but thoughtfully make decisions about which teaching strategies will best meet learners' needs. After determining objectives and learning outcomes, issues of urgency, cost, and efficiency are major concerns. Time frames are often tight and must coincide with new regulations, changes in practice and equipment, or, as in recent years, electronic documentation "go live" dates. Getting the right information to the right employees at the right time and in the right way are critical, particularly in matters of patient safety or regulatory changes.

In hospital environments, it is also common for several education efforts to be underway simultaneously, creating an environment of multiple competing priorities. Employees can be overwhelmed with the amount and frequency of information they are expected to absorb. This can then lead to confusion, frustration, or even learner apathy. Supervisors and managers struggle with schedules and unit budgets, which can become seriously burdened when employees attend class during or in addition to their regular work hours. Make-up sessions for "no show" employees put pressure on educators and further impact the bottom line. For these reasons, online learning options are attractive for the flexibility and scope they offer.

Other factors, however, play into the decision to go online. Depending on the generality of the content and objectives, purchase of an "off the shelf" education product may be a sound option. For material that is hospital specific or unique in nature, such as a pediatric unit's security and visitation strategy, it may be more appropriate to develop online materials in-house. Purchase of ready-made materials may save time, but can be cost-prohibitive depending on licensure policies for multiple users. In-house materials, on the other hand, may save money but can take weeks or months to develop, pilot, and deliver to the learners who need the information. One alternative is to purchase ready-made modules with options for customization, which allows educators to add or edit content to reflect hospital policies and processes.

Other considerations for using online modalities include educator proficiency and comfort with technology, space and instructor availability, stakeholder support and buy-in, learner acceptance of (or resistance to) online learning, and availability of information technology infrastructure and support. In the end, whether online, blended, or more traditional methods are chosen, it is most important that learning objectives, content, teaching strategies, and evaluation methods align to help the learner meet the intended outcomes of the program.

FACILITATORS AND BARRIERS TO USE OF ONLINE LEARNING IN NPD

As stated throughout this chapter, there are recognized facilitators and barriers to the use of online learning in clinical settings. Factors that support the use of online learning include flexibility and convenience of scheduling and the ability to reach a large number of learners in a short period of time. Cost savings are realized through decreased class time, which translates to less "nonproductive" salary dollars, and less need for instructor, space, and printed resources. Learners can easily access online learning resources at their convenience, and LMSs help educators manage registration, routing, and reporting. From a design perspective, materials can be efficiently updated or revised to reflect current standards and practices as changes occur. NPD educators can design modules to appeal to various learning levels and styles, and to adhere to the adult learning principles of relevance, independent learning, and applicability to real life.

Along with these advantages there are understandably certain barriers to successful use of online learning in NPD. From a learner standpoint, barriers may include inadequate computing skills and limited access to computers or courseware. Some learners may demonstrate resistance to a change in how education is delivered, preferring a more traditional classroom or face-to-face approach. From an organizational standpoint a lack of hardware, software, or information technology support for designing and building usable programs may create frustration, administrative bottlenecks, and negative perceptions related to online learning. From an environmental standpoint, noisy stressful work areas, which are commonplace in hospitals, can hamper the online learning experience (Knapp, 2004; Rick, Kearns, & Thompson, 2003).

NPD educators themselves, if not skilled in or supportive of the move to online learning, may inadvertently be barriers to learning. Poorly designed, haphazard online learning materials will quickly lead to learner disengagement and poor learning outcomes. Educators unfamiliar with online teaching strategies should seek out available resources such as SMEs, library personnel, faculty partners, and instructional design experts to ensure that material is appropriate and well conceptualized for online learning. Modules or courses should be piloted and revised as needed before "going live." There are also formal academic courses for NPD educators who desire to improve their online teaching skills. For example, the Institute for Educators at the University of Maryland School of Nursing offers a 3-credit online graduate level course in teaching in online environments, and face-to-face workshops for educators in all settings.

Perhaps a less obvious but important potential barrier is a hesitancy of NPD educators to clearly convey outcomes and return on investment (ROI) of online learning projects. Without compelling data to support new approaches to learning, NPD educators risk losing the opportunity to fully leverage online learning and its many benefits.

MEASUREMENT OF OUTCOMES

According to the ANA Scope and Standards of Practice for NPD (National Nursing Staff Development Organization, 2010, p. 31), educators should "implement a systematic and useful evaluation plan aimed at measuring processes and outcomes that are relevant to the program, learners, and stakeholders." Perhaps due to lack of time and the difficulties of following up with learners in a complex environment, programs are not consistently evaluated beyond the level of a "happy sheet" post-class learner evaluation. NPD educators rigorously track the number of sessions, attendees, and continuing education contact hours related to a particular course. They also collect test scores and learner satisfaction surveys to determine the outcome of classes or courses. However, in order to truly make a case for the benefits of an education effort, and specifically the ROI for online learning strategies, NPD educators are encouraged to fully engage the education process in their approach to program evaluation. Outcomes are defined by the ANA (National Nursing Staff Development Organization, 2010, p. 45) as "something that follows, is the result of, or is the consequence of a project, program, or event." By determining desired outcomes at the outset of a project (i.e., fewer patient falls, decreased catheter infection rates, a 20% shorter turnaround time for medication administration), NPD educators can partner with stakeholders to develop a comprehensive evaluation plan. Ultimately, this approach helps NPD to more accurately demonstrate the value of education. Outcomes related to education can be evaluated via quality improvement and risk management data, chart audits, feedback from participants and stakeholders, and human resources recruitment and retention data, for example (DePew

& Kummeth, 2011). For example, to evaluate the value of a new online fall safety program, NPD educators might compare the cost of new learning technology and software license fees against the cost savings of instructor time, employee salaries, materials and ultimately, a decrease in patient length of stay due to a decrease in falls.

The Kirkpatrick four-level model of program evaluation has been called a "classic in the industry" of NPD (Warren, 2009), and is useful in program evaluation. Its four distinct levels of evaluation help to determine program effectiveness and value (Kirkpatrick & Kirkpatrick, 2006; Bruce 2009). The first level, called *reaction*, assesses whether learners are satisfied with the program from a delivery perspective. Questions may include: Were the instructions clear? Was the content interesting and easily accessible? Was the program length correct? Level two, *learning*, asks if learners achieved what they intended to from the program. Did they achieve stated objectives? Did they learn what they expected to learn? The first two levels can usually be assessed at the time of the training. In an online environment, learners might be asked to complete an evaluation survey before exiting the course or receiving a certificate. *Behavior* is the third level of evaluation in Kirkpatrick's model, and assesses whether the new learning "sticks" over time. In other words, can nurses implement fall precautions and document appropriately 1 month after the training? Can they state fall safety protocols? Level four, *results* or *impact*, looks "down the line" to see if the change has had a positive impact on the system or organization. Educators might use risk management data to determine the number and rate of falls compared to the pre-program data. Because levels three and four take time and require detailed follow-up, they may not be done as consistently as levels one and two. This model is straightforward yet flexible, and could easily be applied to the evaluation of online learning programs in NPD. Use of this or a similar evaluation model to collect evaluation data can add considerable credibility to NPD practice and help solidify the case for incorporation of online learning strategies.

RESEARCH OPPORTUNITIES

There has been remarkable growth in the use of online learning in NPD. To note, a National Nursing Staff Development Organization

(NNSDO) position statement from 2006 did not mention the use of online learning as a staff development tool. Rather, its focus was on online learning as an academic option, and NNSDO supported distance learning as a viable vehicle for learning. By 2009, the Core Curriculum for Staff Development (Bruce, 2009) included an entire chapter on using technology in NPD, and by 2010,the NNSDO Public Policy Agenda (NNSDO, 2010) included a commitment to support education-based research and the use of new pedagogies and technology to connect to nursing practice. The national certification review manual for NPD educators includes use of technology to advance clinical teaching (DePew & Kummeth, 2011).

Examples of online learning and technology-related teaching strategies have been plentiful in the nursing staff development and continuing education literature in recent years as outlined in this chapter. Berger, Topp, Davies, Jones, and Stewart (2009), for example, found that web-based training as compared with lecture, although initially more expensive and time-consuming to create, was more cost effective with large numbers of learners. Sherman, Comer, Putnam, and Freeman (2012) found no significant difference in nurses' learning outcomes or learner satisfaction scores between blended learning and lecture approaches to pharmacology education. Furthermore, Pilcher and Bedford (2011) found that nurses of all ages indicated a willingness to learn using various technological tools. Ease of use, familiarity, convenience, and perceived benefit were the key determinants of their willingness to do so. NPD educators will be wise to incorporate this evidence into their conversations with key stakeholders when lobbying for online education buy-in.

Research evidence on the direct translation of online knowledge to nursing practice is sparse but is gaining attention and momentum, particularly from an ROI perspective. NPD educators and executive stakeholders alike should focus on the "down the line" impact of all educational activities, including online learning. They must question the outcomes this style of learning has on patient care and other measurable clinical outcomes. Studies provide evidence that online formats can be useful in complex clinical environments if barriers are anticipated and addressed. Education provided via an online format can provide a positive learning experience for nurses and other clinicians, yet there are still unrealized or unpublished potential benefits for NPD. Until recently, much evidence about the effectiveness of online learning involved students. Little research existed regarding the impact of an online learning environment on practicing nurses. What evidence there was involved small sample sizes and was not generalizable (Gerkin, Taylor, & Weatherby, 2009). Pressing research priorities for NPD, identified in a nationwide Delphi study, include cost-effective educational and teaching strategies to promote patient safety, nursing competence, and transfer of knowledge in the clinical area (Harper, Asselin, Kurtz, MacArthur, & Perron, 2012). These seem to be areas ripe for the exploration of the benefits of online learning.

FUTURE

The potential role for incorporation of technology and online education by NPD educators in clinical settings is limitless. We can anticipate learners role-playing practice scenarios in virtual clinical units (Wood & McPhee, 2011), online care team chat rooms, mobile preceptor resources, wiki-based case studies, enhanced online partnerships with schools of nursing and other professions, and other applications not yet imagined. Its actual use will evolve at varying paces in different settings, limited by educator experience with online teaching strategies, organizational decisions regarding whether or not online learning is a worthwhile venture, learner acceptance, user sophistication, and technical support to make the online learning experience effective and enjoyable.

The responsibility for demonstrating that online learning strategies can produce a strong ROI in terms of cost and time savings and improved patient and organizational outcomes lies with NDP educators. This must be done via a thoughtful, outcomes-based approach to learning needs assessment, course design, and program evaluation.

REFERENCES

American Heart Association. (2013, January). OnlineAHA.org. Retrieved from http://www.onlineaha.org/index.cfm?fuseaction=main.home

American Nurses Association. (2008). *Professional role competence position statement.* Silver Spring, MD: American Nurses Association.

Berger, J., Topp, R., Davies, L., Jones, J., & Stewart, L. (2009). Comparison of web-based and face to face training concerning patient education within a hopsital system. *Journal for Nurses in Staff Development, 25*(3), 127–134.

Billings, D. M., & Halstead, J. A. (2005). *Teaching in nursing: A guide for faculty* (2nd. ed.). St. Louis, MO: Elsevier Suanders.

Bruce, S. L. (Ed.). (2009). *Core Curriculum for Staff Develoment* (3rd. ed.). Pensacola, FL: National Nursing Staff Development Organization.

Brunt, B. A. (2007). *Competencies for staff educators: Tools to evaluate and enhance nursing professional development.* Marblehead, MA: HCPro, Inc.

Chapman, L. (2006). Improving patient care through work-based learning. *Nursing Standard, 20*(41), 41–45.

DePew, D. D., & Kummeth, P. (2011). *Nursing review and resource manual nursing professional development.* Silver Spring, MD: American Nurses Credentialing Center.

Dumpe, M. L., Kanyok, N., & Hill, K. (2007). Use of an automated learning management system to validate nursing competencies. *Journal for Nurses in Staff Development, 23*(4), 183–185.

Elkind, E. C., Wus, L. R., & Parra, A. J. (2008). The transition of a classroom dysrhythmia course to e-learning. *Journal for Nurses in Staff Development, 24*(6), 286–289.

Elliott, B., & Dillon, C. A. (2012). Online learning—an innovative solution to meeting the challenges of staff education. *Journal for Nurses in Staff Development, 28*(6), 285–287.

Gerkin, K. L., Taylor, R. H., & Weatherby, F. M. (2009). The perception of learning and satsifaction of nurses in the online environment. *Journal for Nurses in Staff Development, 25*(1), E8–E13.

Haggard, A. (2011). Unit inservice classes—are they obsolete? *Journal for Nurses in Staff Development, 27*(6), 301–303.

Harper, M. G., Asselin, M. E., Kurtz, A. C., MacArthur, S. K., & Perron, S. (2012). Research priorities for nursing professional development: A modified e-Delphi study. *Journal for Nurses in Staff Development, 28*(3), 137–142.

Kirkpatrick, D. L., & Kirkpatrick, J. D. (2006). *Evaluating training programs: The four levels* (3rd ed.). San Francisco, CA: Berrett-Koehler.

Klingbeil, C. G., Johnson, N. L., Totka, J. P., & Doyle, L. (2009). How to select the correct education strategy: When not to go online. *Journal for Nurses in Staff Development, 25*(6), 287–291.

Knapp, B. A. (2004). Competency: An essential component of caring in nursing. *Nursing Administration Quarterly, 28*(4), 285–287.

National Nursing Staff Development Organization. (2010). *Nursing Professional Develeopment Scope and Standards of Practice.* Silver Spring, MD: American Nurses Association.

Payne, L. (2012). Electronic classroom: Supporting nursing education. *Journal for Nurses in Staff Development, 6,* 292–293.

Phillips, J. M. (2006). Preparing preceptors through online education. *Journal for Nurses in Staff Development, 22*(3), 150–156.

Pilcher, J. W., & Bedford, L. (2011). Willingness and preferences of nurses related to learning with technology. *Journal for Nurses in Staff Development,* 27(3), E10–E16.

Puetz, B. (1991). Getting ourselves computerized. *Journal for Nurses in Staff Development, 7*(2), 59–60.

Rick, C., Kearns, M. A., & Thompson, N. A. (2003). The reality of virtual learning for nurses in the largest integrated health care system in the nation. *Nursing Administration Quarterly, 27*(1), 41–57.

Shanley, C. (2004). Extending the role of nurses in staff development by combining an organziational change perspective with an individual learner perspective. *Journal for Nurses in Staff Development, 20*(2), 83–89.

Sherman, H., Comer, L., Putnam, L., & Freeman, H. (2012). Blended versus lecture learning: Outcomes for staff development. *Journal for Nurses in Staff Development, 28*(4), 186–190.

University of Maryland School of Nursing. (2013, January). *Teaching in nursing and health professions.* Retrieved from University of Maryland School of Nursing: http://www.nursing.umaryland.edu/academic-programs/grad/certificates/teaching

Warren, J. I. (2009). Program evaluation/return on investment. In S. L. Bruce (Ed.), *Core curriculum for staff development* (3rd. ed., pp. 297–320). Pensacola, FL: National Nursing Staff Development Organization.

Wood, A., & McPhee, C. (2011). Establishing a virtual learning environment: A nursing experience. *The Journal of Continuing Education in Nursing, 42*(11), 510–515.

Wright, D. (1998). *The ultimate guide to competency assessment in health care* (2nd. ed.). Eau Claire, WI: PESI Healthcare, LLC.

Index